*This book is dedicated to all those who have
shared their experiences with me, in whose brave company
I have begun to understand something of what it means
to face the challenge of cancer.*

Praise for *Face to Face with* Cancer:

I found the book immensely practical and also very wide-ranging in the
issues tackled. It is written wisely, sensitively and in an easy-to-understand

to
en

d
ir
o

d
d
n,
at
r!
is
d
d
ie
ts
is

d
ty
d

ie
d
rs
rt

K

face to face with
cancer

Comfort and practical advice
for sufferers and carers

Marion Stroud

A LION BOOK

Copyright © 1988, 1993 and 2004 Marion Stroud
This edition copyright © 2004 Lion Hudson

The author asserts the moral right
to be identified as the author of this work

A Lion Book
an imprint of
Lion Hudson plc
Mayfield House, 256 Banbury Road,
Oxford OX2 7DH, England
www.lionhudson.com
ISBN 0 7459 4854 5

First edition 1988
This edition 2004
10 9 8 7 6 5 4 3 2 1 0

Acknowledgments

Extracts from the following books are reproduced by
permission of the copyright holders: Penny Brohn, *Gentle
Giants*, Century Hutchinson; Elisabeth Kübler-Ross, *To Live
Until We Say Goodbye*, © 1978, Prentice-Hall Inc., Englewood
Cliffs, N.J., USA; Ruth Kopp, *When Someone You Love is
Dying*, © The Zondervan Corporation, USA, extract from
the British edition used by permission of Lion Hudson;
Pat Seed, *One Day at a Time*, William Heinemann Ltd;
David Watson, *Fear No Evil*, Hodder and Stoughton.

A catalogue record for this book is available
from the British Library

Typeset in 10/12 Aldine 721
Printed and bound in Great Britain
by Cox & Wyman Ltd, Reading

Contents

Author's acknowledgments

'No man is an island,' and that is certainly true when it comes to writing a book like this one, based as it is on shared experience. To acknowledge the vital contribution that each individual has made is impossible, for there are so many who have helped and the majority who have talked to me have done so in confidence. Their names and the details of their situation have been changed to protect their privacy. Others have spoken about their experiences quite publicly, and among those I am particularly indebted to Penny Brohn and others who run the Bristol Cancer Help Centre. My thanks are also due to Dr Mary Fenske, who gave me much wise advice from the general practitioner's point of view, and to Sister Trudy Bunday and Mrs Clarissa Robinson, the former home care sister and social worker respectively from the Sue Ryder Home for the continuing care of cancer patients at Moggerhanger. And, finally, this book would never have been written without the practical and prayerful support of my friends, and particularly my husband and family, who have shown incredible patience as we have all weathered the storms of authorship once more.

Foreword

My husband laid the telephone receiver gently back on its cradle and turned to look at me. The loving concern in his eyes made my already churning stomach do a giant-sized leap.

'What did he say?' My lips could hardly be persuaded to shape the words.

'It's not good, I'm afraid.' He paused, obviously trying to find words with which to speak of the unspeakable.

'The surgeon says your father has a tumour of the pancreas. It's inoperable. They can't remove it and there's no other treatment they can give. They have done what they can to make him comfortable, but...' His voice tailed away as he gathered me into his arms.

'How long has he got?' My voice sounded strange and far away; the familiar bedroom felt cold and unwelcoming.

'It's impossible to say for certain, but weeks or months, rather than years.'

'It can't be true... there *must* be something they can do... he didn't look that ill!'

Denial and anger rose up within me. My father had been so full of fun and energy. Certainly he was only a few months away from his seventy-third birthday, but strangers often imagined he was ten years younger. Teachers at my sons' school regularly mistook him for David and Angus's uncle rather than their grandpa, as he helped to ferry the football team to matches in his car, and acted as stand-in umpire for the cricketers. He had been helping in our local Christian bookshop only the day before going into hospital, teasing the younger customers, assisting his 'old ladies' with their heavy bags and distracting restive toddlers as their mothers browsed along the shelves. For him, age was nothing more than a set of figures on a piece of paper. He loved life – and yet, suddenly, sickeningly, a doctor was telling me that my father's life was threatened... that it could well be drawing to a close. The diagnosis was cancer, and that, it seemed, was the end of the matter.

Except, of course, that it wasn't the end... it was the beginning. The beginning of a long hot summer in which my father moved inexorably from diagnosis to death. As I struggled to support both him, and my mother, while juggling with the needs of my husband and five children, two of whom were facing public examinations, it was also the beginning of questions. Factual questions – the whys, what ifs and hows of the physical condition itself. Emotional questions – how did he feel? How did we feel? How does *anyone* feel when faced with a life-threatening disease? How could we all begin to cope, to express our love, face our fears, bear the pain of it all? And spiritual questions – where was God in all this? Did he care? Could he heal miraculously, and if he could... would he? Did a man who had already enjoyed more than the biblically estimated lifespan of threescore years and ten qualify for such special treatment? Should we ask, implore, fight... or simply receive what was to be with open, outstretched hands... quietly accepting... saying in effect, 'Your will be done'? We longed to see a healing, but for whose sake... and would healing begin and end with the physical, or might there be something more?

At that time there was little help for the relatives. When I asked the social worker at our local hospice if there was any literature available to families, she shook her head sadly. 'All I could offer you would be books for the health professionals,' she replied. That might have been of some use for me as a physiotherapist, but would have been of little relevance to my mother, who was struggling with all the medical terminology that tripped so easily off the doctor's tongue.

No one asked us how we were feeling. No one suggested where we might find emotional or practical support. Indeed, when I told the doctor that I wanted to be sure to be with my mother when my father's life drew to a close, he looked at me, surprised. 'Why?' he asked. 'Your parents are both Christians, and so are you. Christians don't fear death. So what is the problem?' The problem was that my parents had been married for forty-five years and my mother was facing the loss of that relationship, with all the anguish that that brings. My sister and I were struggling to come to terms with the possible loss of a beloved father, our children their fun-loving and devoted grandpa. But without realizing it perhaps, the doctor had given me the message that as Christians we were not allowed to grieve, or experience the normal anxieties that beset anyone who is walking with a loved one through a life-threatening illness.

My father's battle with cancer was unusually short. He died twelve weeks after his illness was diagnosed. For the four years after that event, I grieved and tried to make sense of what seemed to be such a waste of a life. I talked to many people who had also come face to face with cancer, and realized that we were not the only relatives who had struggled to know how to love and support the patient in the best possible way. Suddenly the idea came to me. If I could write a book that would help others to do things better, it would be a lasting tribute to the father I loved so much. And so, slowly and painfully, I gathered the information that I would like to have had at my disposal, listened to the stories of others, and eventually a book was written and published. And that, I hoped, would be the end of my cancer experience.

But it was not to be. Sixteen years later I was sitting once more in a doctor's office. This time it was my husband who was the patient, and once again the diagnosis was potentially life-shattering.

'You've got a tumour in your prostate gland,' the surgeon said breezily. 'It's probably not highly malignant, but we'd better get it dealt with.' And so we were back on the treadmill of surgery, hospital visits and uncertainty, and I was confronted again with the questions that I had posed to my contributors all those years ago.

Time has moved on, and so has the approach to and treatment for the various kinds of cancer. But on both occasions, for our family, as for thousands of others before and since, the diagnosis 'cancer' has been a turning point, touching and changing us all. Although we have had to deal with this disease twice, both occasions have heralded an unexpected and uncharted stage in our journey together, with fresh challenges and no easy answers to take with us into the future.

Every individual is unique. So too is every person's reaction to and experience of the disease of cancer. But there are certain basic questions that most of us ask, and need to find the answers to, and sharing them does make a difference. Knowing that others have battled with our sense of isolation, our anger, our hopes and our fears, enables us to walk our own pathway with a greater degree of peace and assurance.

A book is no substitute for people. But whether you are well-supported, or find a listening ear hard to come by, this book is offered as a friend alongside. My hope is that it will lighten the darkness and lessen the loneliness, because everyone who shares their insights and experiences within its pages knows from personal experience what it means to be face to face with cancer.

MARION STROUD

PART ONE:
The initial stage

1 Common questions

'And one thing that I should hardly need to add...' – the physiotherapy tutor paused and fixed us with a stern glare to make sure that we were all still listening – 'There are certain topics that we simply do not discuss while treating our patients: things like sex... politics... religion... and life-threatening disease... er, especially cancer!'

That was many years ago. In the intervening period, politics and religion have definitely lost their place as top conversational taboos, and sex is probably discussed as freely in the wards and treatment rooms of our hospitals as it is on TV chat shows. But 'life-threatening disease... especially cancer'... now, that is another matter entirely.

In a society which prides itself on frankness and fearlessness, and despite the best attempts of many brave people, cancer is still a word that many people regard with almost superstitious dread. They avoid mentioning it, acting as if refusing to say the word will, in some way, keep the disease away. And in spite of the fact that it is the second most common cause of death (after heart and circulatory disease), affecting one in three people in the western world, we are amazingly ignorant about what cancer is, why it occurs, and how it can be dealt with.

All that most of us *think* we know is that the diagnosis of cancer is automatically a death sentence – which is simply not true. It *is* true that every cancer is unique and that the course of the disease and the response to treatment varies from person to person. This means that it is impossible for the doctor – or anyone else – to forecast exactly how any individual will fare. Of course, this can be regarded as bad news, because uncertainty of this kind breeds fear which is very hard to cope with. But it can also be regarded as a reason for hope. After all, if no one is predicting what will happen to me, there is less chance of creating a self-fulfilling prophecy in which I become worse or die within a certain time simply because that is what is expected of me!

Only God knows what next week, next month or next year will bring, and each of us, well or ill, holds only today within our grasp. We can't change the past, but we can considerably darken the present by allowing it to be overshadowed by fears of the future. And even when we are face to face with the negatives of cancer, there are some very real positives. Here are some to hold on to.

o New approaches to the disease and new forms of medicine are being developed all the time, so that it is now realistic to regard forms of cancer such as Hodgkin's disease, acute leukaemia in children, testicular cancer and choriocarcinoma (a very rare cancer of the placenta or afterbirth) as potentially curable.

o Many people are being successfully treated, and although their cancer does not disappear completely, they are able to enjoy active lives living *with* the disease for many years.

o There is a good chance of actually preventing some of the most common cancers by adjustments to our lifestyle. With the explosion of knowledge in the area of genetics, we are now aware of the fact that some people are born with a predisposition to develop certain types of cancer. Tests are available that will indicate the risk of a woman developing breast cancer, for example, when she has a number of close relatives who have had the disease. Such tests are only undertaken after lengthy counselling, however, as some people would find the knowledge that they have a predisposition to the disease impossible to live with. On the other hand, there are those who would prefer to know, and feel empowered by the options that this knowledge would then offer them.

o There *is* information available for those who want it, and things we can do to help ourselves, whether as patients involved in hand-to-hand combat with the disease, or as relatives trying to encourage, support and help in every way that we can. And this is important. It may seem easier, and perhaps even safer, not to grapple with the whys and wherefores of an illness like cancer – to leave all the decisions to the professionals – but this may not be the best way. Robert Tiffany, director of nursing from 1976 to 1993 at the Royal Marsden Hospital in London, says: 'Research has shown that the more knowledgeable patients are about the disease and its treatment and the more they are able to participate in their own care, the better they feel, both physically and emotionally.' And this undoubtedly goes for relatives too.

Of course, there are some questions which do not have satisfactory answers, but there are many others that can be dealt with. We will start with the most basic one of all.

Just what is cancer, anyway?
Although we think of it as one disease, cancer is actually an umbrella term for more than a hundred diseases in which there is uncontrolled growth of body cells.

Normal tissues are made up of individual building-blocks or cells, which are constantly growing and dividing to replace cells that have died. In a healthy body, cells grow and die at roughly the same rate. No one seems quite sure how the cell knows what to do – there is an inborn pattern within each cell like a microscopic computer which is programmed to produce the right size and shape of cell for any particular part of the body Sometimes the 'computer' goes wrong, allowing some cells to change their shape and grow faster than is needed. This results in a 'population explosion', and if these rogue cells are not dealt with by the body's own defences, they form a lump or a tumour. The cellular micro-computer tends to go wrong more often as the body ages, and this is why cancers are more common in older people.

Are all tumours dangerous?
Not all tumours are cancerous or malignant; those that are not are called 'benign'. The main difference between the benign and malignant tumour is that the cells in the benign tumour stay put within the skin or cuticle that surrounds them, and do not spread to other parts of the body. If the abnormal growth causes problems

where it develops, by pressing on the surrounding organs, it will have to be removed. But it is nothing like as troublesome or dangerous as a malignant tumour, whose cells spread through the bloodstream or via the lymphatic system and then form new or secondary tumours in different parts of the body.

Why do some cells become cancerous?
This is a question to which there is no clear-cut answer yet, but there are various clues as to what damages the 'cellular micro-computer' so that it starts sending out the wrong growth and development information.

In the world around us there are cancer-producing substances known as carcinogens. Some are man-made – for example, asbestos and tobacco tar in cigarettes – and some are naturally occurring – for example, radioactive material – which we knowingly or unknowingly absorb into our bodies. Many chemicals, too, are thought to be cancer-producing or carcinogenic. Certain pesticides, some chemical food additives and colourings and a number of industrially-produced dyes are all under suspicion.

In addition to these, some cancerous changes in the reproductive organs are known to be related to hormonal upsets, and viruses are thought to be the trigger factor in one or two cancers – particularly of the cervix (neck of the womb).

Bacteria can also cause problems. Helicobacter can attack the lining of the stomach, causing inflammation which is pre-cancerous. This bacterium can be dealt with by a course of antibiotics, which underlines the fact that it is never wise to ignore persistent indigestion – or any other symptoms that do not go away after a few weeks.

Do carcinogens always produce cancer?
Apparently not. Many people are bombarded by carcinogens over a long period of time and appear to suffer no serious problems, because their bodies' own immune system destroys the cancerous cells before they can form tumours.

Even when tumours have been formed, they are sometimes dealt with by natural means. This was demonstrated by a man who was given someone else's kidney in a transplant operation. The surgeon who was doing the transplant did not notice that the transplanted kidney had a tiny malignant tumour in it. As is usual after such an operation, the patient was given drugs to depress his own immune system and stop his body rejecting the 'foreign' kidney.

All went well with that side of the treatment, but a follow-up chest X-ray showed that there were secondary tumours, typical of those that would spread from a kidney cancer, growing in his lungs. His new kidney was immediately X-rayed and the original tumour was now obvious and growing rapidly.

To save his life, the drugs to suppress his immune system were stopped, and his own natural immunity was allowed to take over the battle. His system promptly rejected the transplanted kidney, so that he had to return to depending on dialysis, but it also destroyed the cancerous growth in his lungs.

Why doesn't the immune system always cope?

This is where we enter an area of heated debate. Some researchers suggest that it is a wearing-down process. If the exposure to carcinogens has gone on for a long time and, in elderly people, the cells are simply getting old, then they are more likely to break down and become cancerous. It is certainly true that the incidence of cancer rises steadily with age.

Others hold firmly to the theory that problems arise when our immune system is suppressed by chronic infection, by a diet high in animal fats and sugars and low in essential vitamins, minerals and dietary fibre, and by prolonged emotional and physical stress.

Stress-related cancers are a very controversial subject, but the theory is supported by many people who link the onset of their own disease with a period of major stress such as a bereavement, redundancy or other crisis. Of course, we all face life-changing stress at one time or another, and by no means everyone going through such a difficult time develops cancer or suffers a heart attack. It would seem that the most important factor in this area is how we actually handle the stress, rather than the stress itself.

Whatever their differences, the experts seem to agree on one thing. Cancer is rarely triggered by a single cause. It is usually a combination of things working together, which just tip the balance of growth, repair and destruction to the negative side.

Having a relative with cancer is a pretty stressful situation. How can we handle it so that we protect ourselves from developing the disease as well?

We have to accept that being face to face with cancer *is* a very stressful experience for the whole family. But we also need to remember that stress can be destructive or constructive according to the way we react to it. There are practical ways of dealing with that stress (we shall explore these in greater detail later on), but the first step is to take as much responsibility for our own health and well-being as we possibly can, by being alert to warning signs and aware of the little things that we can do to help ourselves.

2 Signs and causes

If cancerous tumours cause most trouble when they spread, it follows that to discover the problem early and to get it treated when it is still small and easily dealt with can only be a good thing. It is simpler to do this with some forms of the disease than others, because in some parts of the body it is well hidden, and gives little or no indication of its presence. However, there are certain warning signs which may not indicate anything sinister at all, but should be checked by a doctor, who will *not* think that we are wasting their time.

Warning signs

o A lump or unusual thickening anywhere, but particularly in the breast. Discharge from the nipple or a change in its shape should also be checked.

o A change in normal bowel habits to either persistent diarrhoea or constipation and/or bleeding from the rectum (back passage).

o Blood in the urine, or a need to pass urine frequently or with little warning.

o A sore in the mouth that does not heal.

o Hoarseness of the voice, a persistent cough or difficulty in swallowing.

o Persistent indigestion or vomiting.

o Any bleeding between normal periods or, after the menopause, any bleeding at all, or unusual discharge.

o A sore on the skin that does not heal; a wart or mole that changes colour, shape or size, or bleeds.

Detection

A few tumours can be detected early by simple painless procedures which are becoming more and more readily available. This is known as cancer screening.

o **Chest X-rays** can sometimes detect lung tumours while they are still small.

o **Regular dental check-ups** should ensure that your dentist notices any changes in the soft tissues of the mouth.

o **A cervical smear** involves a few cells being scraped from the neck of the womb and then being examined under the microscope. Any suspicious early changes in the cells can be detected and treated *before* they become cancerous.

o **Breast screening** at its simplest means that a woman examines her own breasts on a regular monthly basis, so that she knows what is normal for her and can quickly detect any changes as soon as they occur. There are leaflets available explaining exactly how to do this (see the list of useful addresses on page 188) and doctors or nurses at family planning or well woman clinics will answer any questions on the technique, as will most doctors.

Some women have naturally 'lumpy' breasts, which makes it difficult for them to decide what is normal and what is not. Other women are considered to be at higher than normal risk because of family history of breast cancer. Both of these groups can be referred to a special breast clinic by their doctor. There a doctor or specially trained nurse will examine the woman once a year and, if necessary, a mammogram may be done. This is a special X-ray of the breast, which is useful for detecting cancers too small to be felt.

o **Blood tests** can be used to detect the presence of prostate and ovarian cancers, although they are not yet 100% accurate.

All these screening tests are simple, painless and widely available, but we often fail to make use of them because we're too busy, too embarrassed, or would rather not think about it.

'Of course,' we say, 'it's a good idea, and I'll get round to it eventually, but at the moment...' Not so. Every step we can take to protect ourselves is worthwhile. So, if these tests are available, use them, and if they are not readily available, ask for them.

Positive action

Doctors are becoming more and more convinced that the risk of contracting the commonest cancers – those of the skin, breast, bowel and lung – can be considerably reduced if we take certain preventive measures.

o **Smoking** Lung cancer has been firmly linked with cigarette smoking; it rarely occurs in non-smokers. Smokers are also more likely to develop cancers of the mouth, pharynx and larynx. This means that giving up the habit, although hard, is the obvious step for smokers to take. Rather alarming statistics have been produced to show that non-smokers who live and work with smokers and so absorb tobacco fumes second-hand also have an increased risk of disease. Vigorous campaigning for smoke-free areas in offices, cinemas, trains, buses and other public places is something we can all do.

o **Diet** 'All the food that I really enjoy,' groaned my friend Susie, 'is either fattening, or likely to give me some ghastly disease! It wouldn't be so bad if all the experts agreed, but they contradict one another at every turn.'

I knew what she meant. There has been a good deal written – and disputed – about what forms a healthy diet, and comparisons between what we eat in the West and what the Japanese or some remote African bush tribe consume are not always very helpful. It may be very reassuring to know that not many Japanese suffer from cancer of the breast and bowel. But then we hear that their diet of raw fish, bracken fern, hot rice-gruel and asbestos-related food additives gives rise to a high risk of stomach cancer. So the dietary exchange does not seem very tempting!

Is it really so important what we eat, especially if cancer is not triggered by one single cause? Many doctors would say that diet is important. Following a high fibre, high in fresh fruit and vegetables, low fat, low sugar eating pattern cannot be guaranteed to prevent us from getting cancer. But there is definite evidence to show that people whose diet is high in animal fat and low in fibre are more prone to bowel cancer. The same eating pattern is likely to result in excessive weight gain – and cancer of the breast and uterus (womb) are more common in overweight women. Given the additional fact that obese people also have a greater tendency to develop diabetes and heart disease, it makes sense to keep our weight down and gradually adapt to a high fibre, low animal fat, low sugar way of eating.

High fibre means:

o more wholemeal bread, fresh fruit and vegetables. Doctors recommend five servings of fruit and vegetables each day.

o less white bread, processed and fast food.

Low animal fat means:

o more pulses, beans, fish and chicken

o less red meat

o more skim milk, low fat cheese and margarine high in polyunsaturates

o fewer full cream dairy products.

Low sugar means:

o less white sugar and sugar-containing foods. (To keep a check on these we need to learn to read labels on tins and packets very carefully.)

This is recommended for healthy living in general, and if it actually helps to prevent disease as well – so much the better. We have nothing to lose and everything to gain.

o **Sun worshipping** There is no doubt that a deep golden tan adds a glow to the body. But our enthusiasm for beautiful bronzing needs to be tempered with wisdom, especially if we have the fair skin type that tends to freckle and to burn rather than to tan. High factor sunscreens (SPF 15 and above), wearing protective clothing and staying in the shade during the hottest part of the day are all important precautions for adults and children alike. Since excessive exposure to the sun increases the risk of skin cancer, including the life-threatening malignant melanoma, it may be better to remain pale and interesting!

This may not sound very appealing, but in this, as in all other steps that we may take to promote good health, it will mean having the courage of our convictions and being prepared to be different if necessary. It all adds up to knowing the facts, counting the cost (in terms of time and thought more often than of money) and taking responsibility for our own well-being.

3 Testing, testing

'If only I knew what was going on I'd feel a lot happier. I feel as if I'm being led blindfold through a maze.'

'One of the worst things about cancer,' said Mary, 'is that it is usually so tucked away inside your body. You can't just look at it and say "that's cancer!" Even the doctor can't be sure, just by your telling him how you feel. I thought that my stomach pains were indigestion... the doctor said that I'd worried myself into having an ulcer, and it wasn't until they did tests in hospital that I knew what the real problem was.'

Mary and her husband felt quite aggrieved about that, but her doctor had not really been at fault. Any number of different diseases may give rise to a similar set of problems, and it is only reasonable to try to eliminate the simpler and more likely causes first. If, after this, the diagnosis is still not certain, the first step the doctor has to take is to locate the source of the trouble, whether it is a tumour or something else. This is usually done by using contrast or plain X-rays, scans, ultrasound, blood tests or direct visual examinations inside the body (endoscopy).

o **X-rays**

The *chest* and *lungs* are simple to deal with – a 'plain X-ray' which needs no special preparation will show those clearly.

The *breast* may need a mammogram which is a special 'plain X-ray' of the breast, which can penetrate the breast tissue at different levels. Often, though, breast tumours are first discovered by being felt by the patient.

If the *stomach* needs to be examined, the patient will probably have to swallow a barium meal. This is a thick white liquid which gradually outlines the gullet, stomach and the upper part of the intestines. Various 'contrast X-ray' pictures will be taken as the mixture passes through the system.

The *large intestine* can be examined by the same method, this time using a barium enema, which is introduced into the body via the back passage.

An *IVP* or intravenous pylogram is a 'contrast X-ray' used to examine the *kidneys* and *bladder*. In this test a liquid is injected into a vein in the forearm and X-ray pictures are taken as it reaches the kidney and bladder.

The *gall bladder* can be looked at in the same way, although in this case the contrast dye is swallowed.

If the *lymphatic system* (which runs parallel to the blood system of the body, carrying the lymphatic fluid which deals with infection) needs to be checked, a dye can be injected into the lymph vessels in the feet, which gradually progresses up the legs and into the abdomen. This is called a lymphangiogram.

o **Scans**

There are two further types of X-ray in the doctor's armoury, and these are the CAT scan and the MRI scan. With the CAT (computerized axial tomography) body scan it is possible to build up a three-dimensional picture of the whole body by taking numerous cross-sectional photographs as the scanner rotates around the patient. The MRI (magnetic resonance imaging) scan uses magnetic waves rather than radiation to form its pictures. Both of these sophisticated machines are now used in most district general hospitals alongside the other methods when contrast or plain X-ray films are not able to give pictures of sufficient detail.

There are other forms of scan in which a tiny amount of radioactive material is swallowed or injected to show up certain areas. *Bones*, *lungs*, the *liver*, *gall bladder*, *kidney* and *thyroid* can all be examined in this way.

o **Ultrasound**

Many of us equate ultrasound scanners with pregnancy, but they do have other uses. Instead of X-rays, very high frequency sound waves are bounced through the body. As these waves send back echoes, the sound pattern they make can be used to build up a picture of the area under examination. This is displayed on a screen, and when the picture is complete, a photograph is taken to provide a permanent record.

o **Blood tests**

A blood test is one of the most common tests in medicine – most of us will have had our blood 'taken' at least once in a lifetime. It is used to diagnose a whole host of disorders, but it is not one of the main tests for cancer, unless a prostate tumour or leukaemia is suspected. A few tumours, however, do produce proteins or 'markers' which appear in the blood – and regular blood tests may be used to give an early warning that these tumours have recurred.

o **Endoscopy**

In recent years a number of instruments have been developed with optical fibres, which enable doctors to see round corners and examine parts of the body that were formerly completely out of reach of the naked eye. These examinations are called *endoscopies* and can be done in:

~the rectum and last part of the large bowel – a *sigmoidoscopy*

~the whole of the large bowel – a *colonoscopy*

~the gullet, stomach and upper bowel – a *gastroscopy*

~the main tubes into the lung – a *bronchoscopy*

~the bladder – a *cystoscopy*.

Most of these tests do not require the patient to be at the hospital for more than a day, and since a sedative is usually given to help relaxation, they are, at the worst, only mildly uncomfortable.

How much will the doctors tell me about these tests?

Most doctors will tell us as much as we want to know. Unfortunately, in the anxiety of the moment, sensible questions often seem to be swept from our minds by a tidal wave of panic, and the doctor may take our silence or hesitation to mean that we don't want to be told.

It is often a good idea to make a list beforehand of things that puzzle or worry us, and if they don't come to mind when we first hear that something serious may be afoot, it is quite permissible to ask for another appointment to get them sorted out.

These are some of the questions that might usefully be raised:

o Why is the test necessary and what is it for?

o How is it done?

o Is any special preparation needed?

o Is it likely to be uncomfortable at the time?

o Are there likely to be any immediate or longer term risks or side effects?

o How long does it take?

o Will it be done as an inpatient or an outpatient?

o If the patient does not have to stay overnight, will they be able to go home immediately (and are they safe to drive), or will they need to be collected?

When they've located the problem – what next?

Even when the doctor has tracked down the area of disease, he cannot tell for certain whether or not it is cancer without taking a small sample of tissue from the affected area. The cells in that tissue can then be looked at under the microscope by the pathologist. This is known as a *biopsy*. Biopsies are usually performed by surgeons, although sometimes they are done by other doctors during the tests which I have described earlier.

For instance, during endoscopy examinations, as well as looking into an organ, the doctor can remove a small piece of tissue with the same instrument. Sometimes a needle is inserted into a lump on or near the surface of the body and a piece of tissue is cut out, or a few drops of fluid withdrawn from inside the tumour. This is commonly done with breast, prostate or skin tumours. It is often possible for a small lump to be removed completely and then examined. If this cannot be done easily, just a portion of it is removed.

What if it is cancer?
If the diagnosis of cancer is positive, the doctor has to ask some questions before planning the course of treatment.

o How large is the tumour and does it involve the normal tissues surrounding it?

o Has the tumour spread to the nearby lymph nodes?

o Has it spread to other organs in other parts of the body?

Depending on the problems that the initial tests (and any succeeding ones that may be thought necessary) reveal, and the answers that they provide to these questions, the doctor will make a treatment plan. He or she has a three-pronged line of attack available in conventional medicine: surgery, radiotherapy and chemotherapy.

o **Surgery**

This is the form of treatment most frequently used. If the tumour is confined to one area and has not spread to distant parts of the body, then it is potentially curable by surgery. It is very important that all of the tumour is removed, and to be on the safe side the surgeon will remove a safety margin of healthy tissue around the growth. He may also remove neighbouring lymph nodes as an added precaution.

Surgery can also be used to make the patient more comfortable, when it is impossible to remove the whole tumour. In this way blockages can be bypassed and pain and sickness relieved.

o **Radiotherapy**

Radiotherapy is the use of a very carefully calculated but concentrated dose of X-rays to destroy cancer cells. It may reduce the size of a tumour or destroy it completely. It is given in small doses over a number of days or weeks. This is because normal cells are also destroyed by radiation and it is important to protect the healthy tissue as much as possible.

Radiotherapy can be used in three main ways:

~to destroy malignant cells in their very early stages (most commonly done for skin cancers).

~to act as a 'back-up' after surgery – destroying any stray cancerous cells that have escaped from the main tumour, and any secondary growths in lymph nodes. Used like this, radiotherapy is rather like soldiers in the rearguard of an army, mopping up pockets of resistance after the main battle has been fought.

~to shrink a tumour that is too widespread to be removed surgically, or to slow down its rate of growth. It is also useful in the relief of pain, particularly when the tumour has formed in a bone. Radiotherapy is also combined with chemotherapy in the treatment of some cancers.

This type of radiation treatment is given by a radiotherapy machine through the skin over the site of the tumour. It does *not* make the patient radioactive. There is, however, another way of treating some tumours with radiotherapy, and this is by implanting radioactive material as close to the cancer as possible within the body.

One fairly new treatment for the early stages of prostate cancer, called *brachytherapy*, involves putting dozens of tiny radioactive seeds directly into the prostate gland where they deliver a measured dose of radiation for the next nine months. These radioactive seeds are not removed, unlike most other forms of radioactive implants which require a short stay in hospital where the patient is nursed in a single room because, while the radioactive implant is in position, they are a minor health hazard to others. However, the implant is always removed at the end of the treatment period, and a full social life can then be resumed immediately.

o **Chemotherapy**

During the First World War a French doctor discovered that soldiers who had been the victims of mustard gas had some distinct changes in the composition of their blood – the numbers of a certain type of blood cell had been considerably reduced.

The observation triggered off the idea of killing cancer cells with drugs, and during the last forty years a number of drugs have been developed which will attack all rapidly-dividing cells. Unfortunately they poison malignant and non-malignant cells alike, and so doctors have to use them with great care. The theory is that the cancer cells will be completely destroyed, whereas the normal tissue will be able to replace itself eventually and so repair any damage.

The advantage of chemotherapy over surgery or radiotherapy is that it can affect the whole body rather than just the local area dealt with by the other two methods of treatment. This is useful when the cancer is widespread.

However, the disadvantage is that the drugs are not choosy about the cells that they attack, and so areas of the body which have normal rapidly-dividing cells – for instance, the bone marrow (making new blood), the bowel, the hair follicles, testes and skin – can be severely affected. Blood composition can be disturbed, hair can fall out and men can become infertile. These, and other problems provoked by the treatment, are known as *side effects*, and the trouble they cause has to be balanced against the good that the drugs may do in curing the cancer.

Some cancers are very responsive to drug therapy and the side effects of the treatment are then considered worth tolerating.

When chemotherapy is decided on as the best form of treatment, either alone or alongside surgery or radiotherapy, the drugs are given in three different ways: by mouth in tablet form, by injection into the muscle or skin, or by injection or drip into a vein.

Treatment may be with one drug only or with a combination of drugs. It varies considerably with the different forms of cancer. Some patients have to stay in hospital for a number of weeks. Others have a three- or four-day course of treatment, with several weeks' break in between each course. And there are others who have to take tablets for quite a prolonged period of time.

We will think about how to help patients through their problems after surgery and the side effects of radiotherapy and chemotherapy a little later on, but before treatment needs to be grappled with, one of the biggest questions of the whole cancer experience has to be faced. How do you come to terms with the diagnosis and accept that the battle is on – that you are actually face to face with cancer?

4 Facing the diagnosis

'The most important interview a doctor will ever have with his patient is that where the diagnosis of cancer is disclosed and treatment options are discussed.'
RAYMOND M. LOWENTHAL

'How did I react to the doctor telling me I had cancer? Shock, shock, *shock*. My stomach seemed to be twisted up in a permanent knot. I just couldn't believe that this was happening to me and yet I was terribly afraid… but for the rest of my family rather than for myself.'

'Knowing that I had cancer was a relief in a way. It was the year before that was really awful. Trying to convince my doctor that I really was ill, and constantly being fobbed off and made to feel neurotic. At least when I knew what I had got to deal with I could get on with the job.'

'My whole world seemed to cave in. It had been a routine operation; I felt so well, and then at my follow-up appointment the surgeon said they'd found this small tumour and that he was afraid I'd need more treatment. It was unreal. I just couldn't take it in. Although it was high summer I felt as cold as ice and just one word was screaming through my mind. *Why?* I drove home like a zombie, vaguely conscious of moving through sun-drenched lanes teeming with life and beauty, yet inside overwhelmed by this awful blackness – supposing there was some tumour left? – it made me feel unclean through and through.'

'How do you feel when someone tells you you have cancer?... The first thought that overwhelmed me at the time was that... I must not let my feelings show... I braced myself, recalled years of admonitions not to "carry on or make a fuss" and replied mildly with something like, "Oh dear, I thought it might be."

'Eavesdropping later on a conversation between my informant and the ward sister I heard that "I had taken it very well." I had not taken it at all well... but I hadn't raged and cried and given him a hard time or adopted the historical Greek style of murdering him on the spot for being the bearer of such grim tidings, so from his point of view things had gone quite well. His management of my crisis consisted of a pat on the hand and the assurance that he was very sorry. I was glad he was very sorry. I was pretty sorry myself. I imagined everyone would be sorry – it seemed inconceivable to me that any reasonable human being wouldn't be very sorry. I didn't think "very sorry" was worth much. That left me with a pat on the hand. Not enough. Not nearly enough... It was a depressingly inadequate encounter.

'It's hard to say accurately what I felt. I only know that the feelings were massive and overwhelming... I can identify with people who describe how frightened they were, but I can identify, too, with the person who admits to anger, panic, even guilt. I felt all those things.'

'The telephone call came five minutes before the children were due to come tumbling in through the front door from school. I stood in the hall and listened to the doctor saying that the biopsy showed a malignancy and that I would have to return to hospital. It was as if he was talking about someone else. All I could think was, "What shall I say to the children? Please God, don't let them notice that there is anything wrong," and a voice inside my head said, "I don't make mistakes." I'm not one of those people who usually hear from God in a dramatic way, but I know this was God speaking because I was wrapped in a cloak of peacefulness that stayed with me right through my treatment and beyond. My best friend wouldn't call me a placid person – my nickname at school was Blitz, so I *know* it came from outside of myself.'

'I told the hospital that I would only accept the chemotherapy treatment that they were offering if they could assure me that there was a good chance of a cure. Otherwise I just wanted to die and get it over quickly.'

'I wasn't told the diagnosis to start with, but my husband was warned by the doctors that I probably had only months to live. Once I knew the situation I was determined to fight – to do everything I could and put up with any treatment that would enable me to live to see my children grow up.'

These are some reactions from just some of the people who have shared their experiences with me. Every individual is unique and each one has their own way of dealing with the situation in which they find themselves. But although the details may vary, almost everyone confessed to a sense of shock (even when the diagnosis was half expected), of wanting to deny that this was happening, and of fear. Cancer is always a disease that we hope will stay away from our door, and if the outlook is not good, then fear naturally increases.

'It's one thing to accept that you have a disease from which you could possibly die,' said Dorothy, 'but it's quite another thing to be told that it's a disease from which you will almost certainly die – barring a miracle. I just fell apart to start with. But I have three things going for me. A doctor who sees me as a whole person, not just a disease, and is honest but always positive. Family and friends who get right behind me and won't *let* me give up. And a belief – faltering at times and I have to keep clawing my way back to it – that God really is in the situation with me.'

o A doctor who is honest and positive.

o A family which is committed and supportive.

o A patient who is determined and has faith in resources beyond his own natural ones.

These three things form a strong fighting force to wage war on cancer. But this effective teamwork does not just happen. It has to be worked for, and is often arrived at slowly, painfully, and with a fair number of stumbles along the way. And one of the first tests is the way in which we handle the diagnosis and its implications.

Who tells what to whom – and when?
The first person to know the results of the tests and biopsy will be the doctor at the hospital. If the investigations have been done on an outpatient basis, the patient will be given an appointment to see the specialist in an outpatients clinic where the results and treatment options will be discussed. Their GP will also be informed by letter or telephone.

Is the patient told straightaway?
Not necessarily. If the patient is recovering after an exploratory operation, it may be a few days before they are in a fit state to ask any questions about their condition, and most doctors like to wait until they are asked before giving information of this sort.

Can the relatives ask for the diagnosis before the patient knows?
Today there is great stress laid on patient confidentiality, and many doctors would consider themselves legally and morally bound to tell the patient first, although of course immediate family can ask to be present, or, if this is not possible, to talk to the doctor themselves at a later date, with the patient's agreement.

What would happen if the relatives wanted to protect the patient from the diagnosis?
Some relatives, fearing that the patient will just give up on the struggle to get better if faced with the news that they have cancer, beg the doctor not to tell. A few want to adopt the 'straight in at the deep end' policy. 'Let's get it over with,' they say, 'and then we can begin to get back to normal.'

Both approaches have very distinct drawbacks.

We need to recognize that many of us hesitate to pass on news of this kind because of our own fears of how *we* will cope, how *we* will be able to support them through it, how *we* will endure watching someone we love coming to terms with such a difficult situation. In other words, it is our own resources we doubt, and need to deal with, as well as any reservations we may have on behalf of the patient.

Fortunately, we usually underestimate the reserves of courage and strength that people possess when faced with a crisis. Yes, there will be anxiety, fear, shock, depression, denial, perhaps even anger and guilt – negative emotions that we spend much of our lives trying to avoid in our happiness-orientated society. But these painful emotions can be worked through together when there is openness and honesty. In the long term we risk paying a far greater price in terms of unhappiness if we deal in concealment and deceit, and doctors are usually very reluctant to travel along that path, for the sake of all concerned.

Having said that, timing *is* important. Being told you have cancer faces you with a crisis that isn't chased away by a few bracing or comforting words. This information needs to be given:

o at the right time – usually when the patient asks or indicates in some other way that they want to know what is wrong. Occasionally they appear to want to stay in ignorance, but most people have a shrewd suspicion what is wrong and welcome a chance to voice their fears. Often a question from the doctor such as, 'Is there anything you want to ask?' will provide the necessary opportunity to put those fears into words.

o in the right way – ideally when the patient is physically and emotionally able to cope

o by the right person – usually the doctor

o in the right amounts – most people can't take it all in at once: always recognizing that it is a life-changing situation which will take time to assimilate and come to terms with.

'I realized eventually,' said Jane, 'that whatever happened, life would never be quite the same again. I was longing to get home and get back to normal, but I know now that I can't expect that. We can't turn the clock back or reverse the changes in my body. So we've got to go forward and find a new kind of normality.'

The medical hierarchy

'I feel as if I'm up against a brick wall!' Bill slammed the phone down and thumped the wall in exasperation. 'I phone the hospital and ask how Mary is, and all I can get from the nurses is "she's comfortable" and "doing as well as can be expected". When I ask what they found when they operated, they say that *they* can't give that kind of information and I'll have to see the doctor. But when I get to the hospital there usually isn't a doctor in sight, and if there is one, I'm not sure if he is the one dealing with Mary. It seems as if they've got a conspiracy of silence!'

A hospital certainly can seem to be a pretty confusing place, and Bill, like many of us, could have done with a who's who to help him find his way through the maze. Some hospitals do issue information booklets to patients, but most of these restrict themselves to telling you about visiting hours and what to bring with you. Few of them appear to realize just how bewildering the medical hierarchy can seem to those not in the know.

In hospitals doctors work in teams, or firms.

The **consultant** is at the top of the ladder. He may be a physician (known as Dr) or a surgeon (known as Mr) and, if the hospital is a centre for teaching medical students, he may be called Professor. He is in charge of the team; his name will be on the chart on the end of the patient's bed or on the board at the clinic. He pays a 'state visit' to the ward two, three or more times a week, with his second-in-command –

the **specialist registrar**, who will be very well qualified and have a number of years' experience in his or her particular field of medicine.

The **senior house officer** will be younger and have less experience, but will still be well qualified. He or she too will accompany the consultant on the 'ward round', but will also be on the ward regularly to supervise the day-to-day care of the patient which will be carried out by –

the **house surgeon** or **house physician**. These doctors will be recently qualified and work long hours, being on the wards on a daily basis, and also have some nights on duty.

So, whom should Bill (and anyone else wanting information) contact?

The house surgeon or physician may well be in the ward during visiting hours, especially if the hospital has 'open visiting' for most of the afternoon and early evening. Ask the staff nurse or sister which houseman is looking after your relative and ask to see that person. They will usually be within the hospital even if they are not in the ward. If your relative has not yet been told the diagnosis, the house surgeon or physician may be able to tell you when the consultant will be talking to them. He may or may not be willing or able to give you more information about what they have found before that happens, but if you feel that you just want to talk to the doctor in charge, you can make a note of the consultant's name and contact their secretary (at the hospital during office hours) to ask for an appointment. If the consultant is available only when you are at work he may be prepared to talk to you over the phone. But obviously a face-to-face interview is better.

A list of questions prepared beforehand will help to prevent your mind going blank. Don't feel awkward about writing the answers down, and checking to make sure that you have understood correctly. Here are some questions that might help.

o What is wrong with my relative?

o What treatment can be offered?

o If surgery has already been done, what has been removed and is this likely to bring about a cure or simply relieve symptoms?

o If surgery is on offer, why is it necessary and what will it accomplish?

o How long will the patient have to stay in hospital afterwards?

o Will any appliance be needed afterwards (e.g. a false breast after mastectomy)?

o Is any further treatment needed – chemotherapy, radiotherapy?

o Is there any alternative to surgery?

o What are the risks involved with the treatment/without it?

o What is the outlook (prognosis)?

These questions may need to be asked more than once. If, as often happens, the initial diagnosis is given to the patient and the relatives at different times, it is very helpful if we can then see the doctor together, so that everyone involved is clear about what has been said. Indeed, many doctors plan to have a second talk, because when we hear the word 'cancer' for the first time our emotions may well take over to such an extent that we simply tune out the rest of the conversation – and then complain that the doctor has not really told us anything!

John and his wife heard about his bowel cancer together, and with his usual managerial calm John interviewed the doctor. He wanted the facts. Details of the immediate treatment and long-term management of his disease were discussed and noted. To all outward appearances John knew what he was facing and was coping well. Back at home a friend asked him how he was feeling.

'Well,' said John. 'I shall be glad when I know a bit more about what I'm up against. The doctors don't seem too sure what is wrong with me.'

John was suffering from selective hearing. In his mind he knew well enough what was wrong, but his emotions were refusing to accept it. He needed gentle repetition and reassurance over a number of weeks before he finally came to terms with the situation.

5 Caring and sharing

'I wanted to help so desperately, and yet in those first weeks after Mike's operation I just didn't know what to say or do. And, so often, what I did say or do seemed to be wrong.'

'I had views about my illness and I needed to have those views acknowledged. It wasn't so important that others accepted what I had to say or even that they agreed with me; but I needed someone to listen and to take *me* into account. But all the supporting cast seemed to have agreed which way the play should be scripted and there wasn't much for the chief actor to say at all.'

'I felt that I had to be the strong one, to support my mother through this crisis, to cope for her... and I knew that if I started talking about the implications of her disease I'd cry and then I was afraid she'd feel even more vulnerable. And that built a wall between us. Then one day she said, "You think I'm going to die, don't you?" and we just cried together. In those few moments the barriers came tumbling down and after that sometimes she supported me, and at others I propped her up. But we were in it *together*.'

'I needed time; time to adjust, to think things through, to get to grips with the situation in my own way. But people kept prodding, asking how I felt – they couldn't seem to understand that I had to grieve alone.'

'I didn't know what to do.'

'I wanted to talk.'

'I felt I must be the strong one.'

'I wanted to be left alone.'

Does any of that sound familiar? There are many variations on the basic scenario, but in the early days after the diagnosis has been given, many of us feel as if we are walking through a minefield without a sniffer dog or mine detector in sight. We feel totally inadequate to deal with a situation which we may well be facing for the first time. And whether, as immediate family, we are in the 'first team' of supporters, or whether we are simply in the reserves – one of the wider circle of family and friends – our reactions can make this time harder or easier for the one who is right at the centre of the situation – the patient.

Patricia Downie, a physiotherapist who worked particularly with cancer patients, wrote in *Oncology for Nurses*:

'Those hoping to help need to be sympathetic without being sentimental, practical without being hard-hearted, to impart hope when all seems black, to be willing to listen, to know when to keep silent and when to seek help. It is not easy... it is learned with experience... and from the example of others who are practised in the art of caring and sharing.'

The art of caring and sharing – that really sums it up. To show that we care and are willing to share – both the burden that another is carrying and our own inner resources. But how can we translate theory into practice most effectively?

Understand the person
It is more important to know the person who has the illness than to know about the illness the person has.

Everyone is different. How vital it is that we acknowledge and accept that fact! And although it is important to be informed about the facts of an illness like cancer, it is far more important to know and try to understand the person who is grappling with the disease, and to allow them the right to handle it in their own way.

There are no pat answers when it comes to estimating how

someone will come to terms with a life crisis. And let us make no mistake: that is precisely what a cancer patient is involved with. Even if a cure is expected, at the time of diagnosis, they are facing the possibility of loss on a grand scale.

There is certainly a present *loss of health*.

There is a *loss of role*: they are no longer able to do what they would normally do at home or at work.

There is a *loss of control*: doctors and others are telling the person what is best for them.

And there is a possible *loss of life*.

This is not a situation that any of us would choose.

The experience of loss is likely to cause depression and anxiety to a greater or lesser degree. How much a person suffers in this way depends on their natural temperament, their own inner resources, and the baggage – past experiences and present problems (other than the illness) – that they bring with them into the situation. It does not *have* to happen, but if it does, we should not be surprised – it is not a sign of failure on their part or ours, but a normal human reaction. It needs to be recognized and accepted rather than ignored, and the patient needs to be loved through it rather than jollied out of it.

One wise counsellor defined empathy as 'your pain in my heart', and this is what caring really involves. It means sharing another's pain; moving into their space with them – not to criticize or condemn, but to identify with them and to be lovingly available as and when they feel that they need us, and not according to our timetable.

Recognize the stages of grief

Cancer is a life-threatening disease, and it makes those suffering from it much more aware of the reality of death, even in the early stages of their illness. As one person put it: 'I suddenly realized that the diagnosis of cancer was not necessarily my appointment with death. But it was that diagnosis that made me aware that every human being does have that death appointment sooner or later.'

Dr Elisabeth Kübler-Ross, a Swiss-born psychiatrist living in America, has pioneered a very positive approach to the care and support of those who are in this position. She has described people's emotional response to dying as moving through five stages. People do not necessarily wait until the final period of their illness before experiencing these emotions – the possibility of death is enough to trigger them. Nor do they always pass through them all, or work through them in the same order. But it is helpful to know what they are, so that if and when they occur, we are not taken by surprise.

o **The denial stage**: 'This can't be happening to me.' This is a very common reaction to any unpleasant news or situation, and we have seen that most people respond in that way when first faced with the diagnosis of cancer. The denial acts like a buffer, creating a safe area where we can stop for a while and adjust to the situation. Given time, most people move on to acknowledge the reality of what is happening, although they may need a little help to do so.

Take John, for instance, the patient who had been told the diagnosis and not 'heard' it. He needed to be reminded of what had been said, whenever he raised the issue, in a matter-of-fact way and without blame or criticism for not having heard it the first (or second or third) time.

Mary had 'heard' her diagnosis, but denied it by insisting that the doctor must be wrong. She demanded a second opinion and then a third. Her husband went along with her denial at first, asking for the additional consultations and going with her to see the doctors. But when her refusal to accept the diagnosis put her at risk because she was delaying treatment, he decided to face her with the evidence and the dangers of her denial. It was only then that she was able to let it go.

Occasionally people hang on to their denial while still accepting the treatment offered, like the old lady who was being cared for in a hospice during the final stage of her illness.

'I can't think why I'm here,' she confided to a nurse. 'Everyone else has cancer except me.' And she apparently remained genuinely convinced that this was the case until her dying day. The nurse did not try to argue with her. She knew that the patient had had the true situation explained to her and she recognized that denial was this individual's way of handling the situation. She was not endangering herself by doing so, and her right to cope with her illness in the way that was right for her was respected.

o **The anger stage**: 'Why me?' This is one of the commonest
questions that a doctor is asked at the time of diagnosis. 'Why
have I got cancer? Why me?' In fact, many patients seem to be
more concerned about *why* they have developed the tumour than
what its implications are.

Of course, the question may be a genuine request for
information, but it is more often an expression of underlying
anger and grief. It is natural, when faced with an intolerable
situation, to look for someone to blame. Some people blame
themselves, berating themselves with questions like:

'Why didn't I give up smoking?'

'Why didn't I examine my breasts more regularly?'

Others blame the doctor. 'If he had listened to me more
carefully he would have recognized the problem sooner. But my
doctor is always in such a hurry.'

Many blame God, but try to suppress their anger because they
feel obliged to keep up a facade.

Kaye, a nurse and a vicar's wife, was horrified to discover her
reaction to her illness.

'I was bitterly, furiously angry when the diagnosis was
confirmed. I had spent my life giving out to other people, so why,
I asked myself (because I dared not ask anyone else – it would
have sounded too unspiritual), should God allow this to happen
to me? What had I done to deserve it? Then one half of me began
to feel guilty for having such thoughts, while the other half felt
totally justified for feeling so furious. On the surface I was coping,
being brave, giving the right answers, but underneath I was like
a volcano just waiting to erupt.'

Fortunately, someone came along who sensed her inner
turmoil and helped Kaye to express how she was feeling.

'The chaplain came to see me and asked me how I felt. Of
course, I gave him my standard answer, but then he said, "Do
you ever wonder what God is doing in all this?"

'I let him know exactly what I wondered! He didn't seem
shocked and he didn't argue. He just listened and then he said,
"I don't have any answers as to 'why?' Maybe God will show you
one day, maybe he won't. But perhaps that is the wrong question.
Have you thought of asking 'what?' What is God wanting to do

in my life through this illness? Ask him that, and don't be afraid to tell him how confused, angry and hurt you feel. He knows anyway."

'It wasn't what I wanted to hear. But just telling someone was such a blessed relief that I did what he said. And gradually the anger went and I began to look at the whole situation differently.'

Like Kaye, many people suppress their anger and often refuse to admit that it even exists because, since childhood, they have been taught that 'nice people don't get cross' or variations on that theme. And yet anger is not necessarily wrong, and expressing it in the right way can be an important part of the healing process. Elisabeth Kübler-Ross says: 'Those who have not been able to externalize their fears and frustrations, their guilts and unfinished business remain stuck in them. Those who have had the courage to scream and rage, if necessary, to question God, to share their pain... are the ones whose faces were peaceful and radiant... in the final days of their earthly existence.'

So firmly does she believe that it is important to discharge anger that she often gives her patients or their families a short piece of rubber hose. When the emotional temperature reaches simmering point, they can express their feelings of rage and frustration privately by beating a mattress or cushion with the hose, instead of lashing out verbally or physically at another person.

o **The bargaining stage**: 'Yes – but not yet.' Offering one thing in exchange for another is something that we do all the time; even quite small children learn to drive a hard bargain with each other. So it is not surprising that people bring those negotiating techniques into their handling of serious illness. A bargain in this situation is often offered to the doctor in relation to gaining time. 'If you can help me to stay well for long enough to organize my daughter's wedding I shan't ask for anything more.' 'I'll have any treatment that you suggest if you can assure me it will allow me to live to see my children finish school.'

Having a strong motive for staying well has a very positive influence on the course of an illness. Someone who has a purpose for living often seems to cope better with anxiety – and so will be likely to suffer less from sleeplessness, pain and a poor appetite. Of course, this is just what a doctor wants for his patients, and he will do all in his power to fulfil his side of the bargain. But the final outcome is not completely in his hands, which may be why most people, whether they have a strong personal faith or a very flickering glimmer of belief, try to make a bargain with God.

'I wrapped it up in very holy language, I suppose,' said Stella. 'I begged God to heal me so that I could serve him even more – and I was already very busy in the church. I promised that I would make sure that he would get the praise for my healing – I'd let everyone know that it was a miracle. I meant it, I really did, but underneath all that, *I* knew (and *he* knew) that my main motive for wanting to get well was to stay with my family.'

George had more of a nodding acquaintance with God:

'I prayed now and then, if things were difficult with the business. I went to church at Christmas – that sort of thing. But when I had to face the fact that I might not have much time left I thought I'd better get myself sorted out. So I told God that if he would make me well – with or without the help of doctors, I wasn't fussy – I would go to church regularly and give them a bit of financial help to put up the new building they needed.'

Much to George's surprise, he was warmly welcomed at church, but his offer of financial help was shelved for the time being at the minister's request.

'He said that God wanted me, not my money, and that I couldn't buy my healing any more than I could buy forgiveness. I didn't like it at first, but I thought it over and I've come to see that if he loves me, he'll do what is best for me anyway. I'm not free of the cancer yet, but I keep praying. And I'm helping with that new building – no strings attached!'

o **The depression stage**: We have already seen that when anyone has to face up to loss, there will inevitably be mourning for what has been, or what may be, taken away. This sadness will ebb and flow throughout the course of an illness. The full extent of the loss may not have been experienced yet, but the anticipation can be as painful as the real thing. Many of us find it hard to cope with our own sadness, and even harder to see a loved one grieving. We feel at a loss to know what to do or say, but that does not matter because it is often better to say very little. I asked people with cancer what helped them through this stage of their illness – and what did not.

'I wanted someone to acknowledge how I was feeling – to agree that it was horrible to be faced with cancer. At that moment I didn't *want* to be cheered up and told that everything was going to be fine.'

'I needed permission to cry – and to rage and to shout – until I felt better. One person did this for me. She didn't offer me a handkerchief when her shoulder was soaked through and *she* had had enough. She waited until I was ready to stop before mopping me up.'

'Talking wasn't really the most important thing. It was having people there who could be quiet, hold my hand and assure me that I wasn't on my own in the darkness. They were there and I knew they wouldn't leave me – that's what made the difference.'

'I must have been impossible to visit. I didn't want to be told that I was a fraud because I looked so well – but I certainly didn't want to hear that I looked poorly! I didn't want to hear all my visitor's troubles – and yet I wanted to know what was going on in the world outside. Sometimes I wanted to talk about my illness and at others 1 couldn't bear to mention it. What I needed most were the two or three people with whom I didn't *have* to cover up – who could accept how I was feeling on any particular occasion without being shocked or getting upset because I wasn't coping. And who never gave up or stopped hoping – and wouldn't let me do so either.'

o **The acceptance stage**: This is the final stage of the grieving process, and like all the others it is often grasped, lost sight of for a while, and then experienced more fully.

Acceptance does not mean giving up the struggle, but coming to terms with the facts.

It does not mean leaving all the responsibility to someone else, but being ready to face up to the situation oneself.

It does not mean constantly dwelling on an uncertain future, but concentrating on dealing with the joys and sorrows of today.

That is the ideal, although not everyone will be able to do it for all or even part of the time. It is not a goal for the patients alone. The first team supporters also have to come to a point of acceptance if they are to form an effective fighting force with the patient and doctors. So, having given some thought to the patient's needs and reactions, let's explore how their supporters can meet the demands on resources that being face to face with cancer will bring.

6 Understanding ourselves

'Your father has cancer.' Those four simple words hit me like a douche of icy water. My most vivid memory of the weekend that followed is of feeling cold... terribly cold, in spite of the spring sunshine outside and the centrally-heated house. Food seemed to stick in my throat, and the little that I did manage to eat shot straight through me. Looking back I understand what did not occur to me then – that my body was simply reacting physically to the shock my mind and emotions were experiencing.

And so it is with us all. We may experience those emotions, which are part and parcel of grief, in different ways (emotional ups and downs of any kind have always gone straight to my stomach), but experience them we will. Of course, our closeness to the patient will have a bearing on the degree to which a diagnosis of cancer will affect us. It will obviously impinge more forcibly on the life of a parent, husband, wife or older child than on that of a casual acquaintance. But I am assuming that if you are reading this book you are closely involved, one of the first team supporters – a part of the family or a close friend. And what we often fail to grasp (perhaps because no one thinks to warn us) is that there will be things other than practical matters to be sorted out for ourselves, before we can really offer the patient the kind of support that we long to give.

We need to understand a number of things.

Baggage from the past
We walk into this crisis situation carrying our own luggage. What kind of a picture does that statement conjure up in your mind?

I visualized a stream of refugees fleeing from some invading army, carrying as many of their possessions as they could possibly cling to. That may not be an entirely accurate illustration of what we do, but it is not completely off-beam. For just as the way the patient faces up to his illness is influenced by his experiences earlier in life, so it is with the support team.

In the four months before my father's illness was diagnosed, two other close relatives had died from cancer, and my parents' dog had had to be 'put to sleep' because of a canine form of the disease. So the word cancer had a pretty bad press in our house, and I could be said to have been carrying a suitcase labelled 'people die from cancer'.

I also had a rather old and shabby bag, filled with my experiences as a physiotherapist treating people who were adapting to artificial limbs after amputations for bone cancer. I had given breathing and other exercises to patients after surgery for lung and breast cancer too. The label on that bag might have been 'cancer means major operations'.

And then there was some current luggage, labelled 'the children need you,' because my two oldest sons were facing major school examinations that summer.

This was just some of the baggage that *I* carried into our family's experience of cancer, and of course this influenced the way in which I coped with the situation. If I had realized this at the time, it would have helped me to understand my emotions and reactions better, even though I could not have altered anything.

The threat of loss
We, too, will experience the stages of grief, because of the loss that threatens *us*.

We have already thought about the way in which the patient moves through the stages of denial, anger, bargaining and depression until he finally accepts his illness. And once we know that it *may* happen, it is easy to spot it when it does happen. But we may be rather slower to recognize that those close to the patient will also be facing the threat of loss and change in a number of areas of their lives.

There is *loss of security*: life is no longer following its normal pattern, and the future is full of question marks.

There is *loss of control*: decision-making for the well-being of the patient is at least partially removed from the family and taken over by 'experts'.

There is *loss of support*: if the patient has been the strong, supportive member of the partnership or family group, for a time at least, the supporter becomes the supported. This is often very hard for both parties initially. The less dominant partner may well resent being forced to take over a role they neither want nor feel equipped to cope with (and then feels guilty for feeling resentful). And the patient may feel humiliated and useless because he or she can no longer carry on as usual.

There is *loss of relationship*: the fear that the patient may not recover poses a threat to the very existence of the relationship.

And so it is hardly surprising that we will have our own grief to work through. Many people feel that they have failed if they become tearful, angry, anxious or depressed when they want to be cheerful, loving, peaceful and positive for the sake of the patient. But we all need to understand that in this situation we are not being failures – we are being human. That does not mean our reactions do not matter. They do, and they need to be shared.

Sometimes it is right to share them with the patient. Crying together can break down barriers and help us to be real with one another. Sharing our anxiety about situations at home and asking for their advice can help those who are ill to feel that they still have a contribution to make and a role to play. But in the stage of the illness when the patient is still coming to terms with the diagnosis and coping with initial treatment, that kind of sharing needs to be done wisely and with care.

It is at this point that it is particularly helpful to have our own group of supporters – the reserve team, if you like – who will listen to *us* and give *us* practical and emotional help. Being one step removed from the situation and less emotionally involved, it is easier for them to see things more clearly and to be sympathetic, practical and positive. Not everyone has these gifts to offer, but if we are fortunate enough to have friends like this, we should accept help gratefully and forget about 'coping' and 'keeping a stiff upper lip'. If we do not have this kind of support from our friends, we should not be ashamed to seek it from professionals. More and more people are being trained to help the cancer patient and his or her family, and the doctor will be able to supply the names of local contacts. There are also national bodies that can help (see the list of useful addresses on page 188).

Facing reality

The kind of relationships that existed before cancer is discovered will still exist after the diagnosis is given.

Developing cancer does not make the sufferer a saint overnight, and a cancer patient's relative or close friend is not automatically issued with wings and a halo.

Margo and Don were having counselling to help them sort out their marriage difficulties *before* Margo's cancer was discovered, and they needed even more skilled help afterwards. This shocked Margo's parents, which was really quite illogical: after all, they had the same old problems plus some extra ones to contend with!

So we need to be realistic. I am not suggesting that the experience of having cancer does not change people – it does, and quite often brings a totally new and positive dimension to the lives of all those involved. However, that change takes place gradually. We may well have an ideal towards which we want to work, but we have to start with the raw material of the relationship we already have. And we need to realize that there is no stereotype which has to be achieved, no set of rules that has to be obeyed, in order to be a 'good' patient or a 'successful and caring' relative. Each of us needs to know and accept our own capabilities and limitations and work within them.

Accepting limitations

We do not have to carry out the whole burden of care.

In the emotional turmoil of first discovering that someone we love has cancer, it is easy to feel that we are responsible to cope at all times and to supply their every need. This is nonsense. While it is true that in a loving relationship we will want to do all that we can, it is not humanly possible to be 'everything' to another person. It may hurt our pride to admit it, but when we do, it rolls a tremendous weight from our shoulders.

We need to accept that although we can, with God's help, be a channel for his love in the situation and know resources far beyond those we possess naturally, to be totally loving, completely understanding, all-wise, all-knowing, endlessly supportive and absolutely tireless is something only God can be. And he can and will be that to patient and relatives alike. However, he often demonstrates those qualities to us in practical ways through other people.

It is like a safety net. The anchor ropes at either end hold the whole thing safely, securely and in position. They could be a picture of God's part in the proceedings. The outside ropes which form the firm edge and give the whole net its shape are like the closest family, absolutely vital. But that outside rope is far too short to fill in the central fabric of the net. A whole extra network is needed for that. In the case of the support team they can be ropes of different lengths, different colours and even different thicknesses – friends come in all shapes and sizes, but each has an important and unique contribution to make.

Other people

We must allow others to cope with the situation in their own way.

Not everyone will want, or be able, to form a major part of the safety net. We may find people, even within the family, from whom we might have expected a good deal of support who are unable to offer much.

Sometimes the reason may be fairly obvious. Tina's ten-year-old daughter had had juvenile rheumatoid arthritis since she was six, and Tina had daily exercises to carry out with her at home, as well as twice-weekly visits to the hospital for physiotherapy. Her husband had been made redundant the year before and was struggling to start his own business with Tina's help when his mother's bowel cancer was discovered. Tina was very concerned about her mother-in-law, but she felt that every ounce of her physical and emotional energy was already spoken for, and she was unable to do more than make a daily telephone call and a weekly visit.

Other reasons may be less easy to understand. Anne lived two hundred miles away from her mother, whereas her sister Kate still had her home in the small town in which they had been brought up. But when their mother developed a brain tumour, it was Anne who was expected to travel long distances to see the consultant, visit her mother and nurse her in the final stages of her illness. Kate insisted that she could not take time off work, and in any case was 'hopeless with sick people', so although she looked after her mother's financial affairs she gave little other practical or emotional help.

What should we do if we are faced with this kind of situation?

We can deal with it in one of three ways. The ideal is to have an open and honest discussion about what contribution each person involved is willing and able to make. If this does not happen, or if the offers made are not very satisfactory, we can try to understand why others are reacting in the way that they are, allow them to deal with things in their own way, and cheerfully accept the level of help that they *are* able to give. Or we can become resentful and angry.

The first two courses of action give us a platform on which to build; the third will be like a corrosive acid, distorting and destroying relationships long after the immediate crisis is over and forgotten.

Helpful advice

We will need to trust our own judgment.

People love to give advice, and since much of that advice will be based on hearsay, or half-understood chunks of popular medicine dispensed by the television or magazines, it can be very confusing and unsettling, especially when one piece seems to contradict another.

David Watson was well known as an outstanding Christian teacher when he developed bowel cancer. After he came home from hospital (with a very poor prognosis because the disease had spread to his liver), he gave a radio interview in which he spoke very frankly about his battle with the disease. Partly as a result of this, he and his wife, Anne, were bombarded with books and articles on cures for cancer, sent by well-meaning friends and strangers alike. He wrote about this in his book *Fear No Evil*.

'Many of the books suggested special diets, and these often differed from one another, which we found most confusing... together they gave Anne the gut feeling that my life was in her hands... As I saw her becoming more and more tense with each new book arriving, I realized that any marginal benefit emerging from a better diet would be cancelled out immediately by the marked increase of tensions in our lives. Although I do not doubt that some people can benefit from a strict diet, and perhaps even overcome cancer in this way, we felt that simple adjustments, such as an increase in fruit and raw vegetables and a general avoidance of unnecessary toxins was all that we could handle peacefully.'

Few of us will be likely to be the subject of that degree of public concern and attention, but we will all have to be prepared to choose our course carefully and stick to it, even if we are faced with some opposition.

A vital faith
God is still there in the darkness.

Many people who have shared their experience of the cancer crisis have been insistent that the whole struggle would have been impossible without their 'sure and certain hope' in the love and faithfulness of God. But having a vital faith does make demands upon us. If you believe that this life is all there is, and see yourself as entirely responsible for your own fate, you are at least spared the questions about why a loving God should allow suffering, whether he can and will heal miraculously today, and other theological conundrums. But if recent opinion polls are to be believed, only a very small percentage of the population is in that position. The rest of us have some belief in God, ranging from hazy to very clear. And that belief often has to be reconsidered and reaffirmed as it faces the challenge of life-threatening disease. We shall consider the questions of suffering and healing a little later on, but there are certain very practical problems which need to be mentioned at this point.

Mary had always been a very disciplined and devout person and did her best to make herself available to help others in need. But when her husband developed cancer she found it almost impossible to pray, read her Bible, attend church regularly, or handle any other problems but her own. She was so worn out with visiting the hospital and coping with her own family and part-time job that if she sat down she fell asleep. This worried her. She was half afraid that God might forget her if she appeared to have forgotten him.

Tom believed that Christians should be peaceful and trusting whatever the situation, and so when he felt anxious and fearful about his brother's illness he considered himself to be a failure. Not wanting others to know how he was letting the side down, he hid behind a cheerful facade, insisting that all would be well – but weeping inside.

Sally felt that she was suffering from a double bereavement.

'As I faced the fact that my father was dying, a grey depression wrapped itself around me like a stifling fog. I was frightened as well as depressed. Not only was I facing the loss of my earthly father, but my Heavenly Father seemed to have moved out of my life as well. What few prayers I could pray seemed to bounce back at me off the ceiling, and I had no sense of God's reality or nearness any more. At first I wondered what I had done wrong. Then I began to get angry and question whether my faith had been a giant hoax all along.'

Mary, Tom and Sally all had lessons to learn – and so will the rest of us, as we work out our faith in relation to this new experience.

The nature of God's love

God loves us as we are, and for what we are, not for our religious observances or good deeds.

The psalmist put it this way: 'As a father has compassion on his children, so the Lord has compassion on those who fear him; for he knows how we are formed, he remembers that we are dust.'

Mary began to understand that it was both possible and acceptable to bring her problems to God at any time, in brief conversational prayers rather than the more formal approach that she had used before. As she did this her faith developed into a living relationship rather than a formal ritual. She also found herself able to relax and rest in the fact that others could pray for her when she could not pray at length for herself. The supporter could become the supported for a while, and no one would think any the less of her.

The peace of God

It is possible for Christians to know the 'peace that passes understanding', but that does not mean they should never experience, or admit to, grief or fear.

The peace of God is given in the middle of the storm and not instead of it. Tom only began to discover this peace when in desperation he allowed his mask to slip, admitted his anxiety to God and shared the burden of it with trusted friends. Much to his surprise, he was not criticized or condemned but loved, prayed for and taken care of in the practical ways that he and his family so desperately needed and yet had been ashamed to admit.

Asking questions

God does not condemn us for our questioning.

The desolation that Sally felt is by no means an unheard-of occurrence. Job is the Bible character best known for his struggle to make sense of suffering in the light of God's character. And there have been many thousands of people since who have experienced what people in earlier centuries have called the 'dark night of the soul', when God seems far away and uncaring.

Why does it happen? Is it something we bring on ourselves? Sometimes it is. If we persistently nurse bitterness and resentment in our hearts, or deliberately do what we know to be wrong, we soon sense a barrier between ourselves and God. King David wrote in the Psalms: 'If I had cherished sin in my heart, the Lord would not have listened.'

Jesus himself knew a sense of abandonment beyond anything we can feel as he took on himself the crushing weight of human sin during the crucifixion. In total desolation he cried out, 'My God, my God, why have you forsaken me?' He was truly cut off from God, so that no one need ever again face that ultimate loneliness.

But our own 'dark night of the soul' is less often a correction than God's way of refining and toughening our faith. Idling along on a level road does little to build up our physical stamina – it is only when muscles are asked to overcome resistance and do more work than they have done before that they develop strength and endurance. And so it is with faith. If there are no challenges to face or problems to overcome, faith and trust will have little reason to grow and endure.

A small child needs a caring adult to hold his hand and keep him safe as he walks along a busy road. As he gets older, that steadying hand is gradually withdrawn, the adult steps into the background and the child goes on by himself. We would be very concerned if an older teenager was afraid to walk alone. And so it is with faith. As part of the maturing process, God sometimes withdraws the *sense* of his presence, so that we learn to live spiritually by depending on faith and not on feelings.

But sometimes we prefer to react like angry children when things do not go our way. Just as a child in a temper often pushes away the one thing he really wants most – the loving arms of his mother – so we can cry out to God and yet almost refuse to receive his comfort if it is not offered in the form in which we want it. There is only one solution, and that is to bring the whole misery of our situation, the questions and the anger to God, and wait for his answer.

Ruth Kopp, a doctor who specialized in the care of cancer patients, wrote:

'I do not believe that God expects us to accept our difficult situations automatically and without question. When we ask our questions he will respond, although he may not always give us direct answers. In some cases he will make all or part of his purpose behind the situation clear... the rest of the time we must be content to know that he *has* a purpose. We must trust him in the light of what we already know and in the light of the new knowledge of him that we acquire while in the midst of our trouble. Although God may not satisfy our desire to understand, I am confident that he will always satisfy our need for his presence and his love. When we need him, cry out to him and wait for him, we *shall* find him.'

And this does not apply only to those who have a sure and steady faith. God has promised that anyone who genuinely seeks him will indeed find him.

7 Patients are people

'A cancer patient isn't merely an individual with a diseased body; he is above all a person with a thinking mind and a stirring soul. He has attitudes and aptitudes, interests and instincts, hopes and dreams which are all affected by his condition.'
ROBERT TIFFANY

There's more to being a patient than just being patient.

When I was a child, hospitals fascinated me. I loved the smell, the hustle and bustle as patients and staff were either helped or hurried from one place to another, and the sense of being in a little world that was self-contained and full of drama. However, I suspect that I was – and am – very much in the minority. Most people find a hospital rather a threatening place, at least at first. There may be a sense of relief that something is being done about the illness, but there is also a mixed bag of more negative emotions.

'The day before I went into hospital I had an important job to do. I was secure in my own world, in control, with a full diary. I had secretaries to cope with the small details of my working life, while I made decisions – decisions which would affect the way others lived and money was spent. Twenty-four hours later I walked into the ward and became a totally different species – a patient. Taking off my clothes had a greater significance to me than simply carrying out the nurse's request.

'I felt stripped of everything. Instead of being in charge, busy, under pressure certainly but enjoying it, I was faced with empty hours sitting and waiting for things to happen, and for others to make decisions on my behalf. I saw my wife leave the ward carrying my clothes and I felt a tremendous sense of loss – ridiculous but very real!'

This sense of vulnerability and anxiety is not just caused by ignorance of what lies ahead. Hospitalized members of the medical profession often feel just the same.

'I was beginning to wake early each morning, and in the long pre-dawn darkness exaggerated dread of the operation filled my mind. It was always my first thought and almost impossible to shake off. I am a trained nurse, so why should I be so full of apprehension? Was it because... the thought of being a patient went greatly against the grain? My mind began to visualize every detail of what would lie ahead: admission to the ward, physical examinations, preparation for surgery, the actual operation... I found myself going on to imagine what waking up afterwards would be like; the pain, the drip, the embarrassing total dependence upon others. My mind stopped there... I didn't think much about recovery or the joy of returning home. The dread side of it all was too prominent.'

This sense of being dependent on others and 'out of control' is something that a number of patients find difficult. It is not helped by the 'them and us' attitude which tends to exist between the medical staff and those they are caring for. Nurses are often working under pressure and, although they give excellent physical care, can appear to be too busy to chat and to give emotional support. Doctors come and go in the wards and are often regarded with a reverence akin to awe by the patient, which makes real communication difficult.

In her study *Human Relations and Hospital Care*, Ann Cartwright surveyed a number of patients and asked them who their main informants about their condition were. Forty-six per cent specified one or other of the doctors on the team, and yet fifteen per cent did not even know the doctor's name. Of those who did know who was treating them, only seven per cent of the patients said that the doctor introduced himself, and one per cent asked him outright who he was. The majority of the rest gained their knowledge from the nursing staff or other patients. Hardly a good basis for effective teamwork!

People seem to fall into two categories as patients. First, there are the 'passive receptors', who seem to feel that, once in hospital:

o they have handed over all responsibility for their health to others

o they must do nothing without permission

o they must ask no questions

o they must accept what they are told

o they must conform meekly to the hospital routine.

They are often considered ideal patients by the kind of staff who like beds to be immaculate, locker tops uncluttered and patients lying tidily in bed, preferably to attention!

Then there are the 'active initiators', who:

o need to maintain control over their destiny – at least to the extent of understanding what is happening to them. So they want to know what, why, how, where and when – and if they do not get satisfactory answers the first time, they ask again!

o handle their anxiety about the unfamiliar by asking detailed questions about the technical side of their treatment

o do not suffer in silence, but want to share with someone how they feel about their illness.

All this takes time, and may not fit in with the streamlined organization of hospital routine. So these individuals are sometimes labelled 'difficult' patients, but we should not let this put us off asking questions or wanting to be involved with decision-making as far as we can. Current medical thinking is that 'bolshy patients do best,' and that teamwork is important. So if a few members of the old school have not discovered that yet, that is their problem, not ours.

One thing we should be aware of, though. Some patients prefer to take the passive role – at least initially. It is all that they feel that they can cope with, and as such it is right for them. If we as relatives want to be more active, we can ask questions on our own behalf and encourage patients *gently* by sharing our information and giving them as much opportunity as possible to be involved. But we should never try to force them into a mould that does not fit. Even if bolshy patients *do* do best, that strength, determination and willingness to take responsibility has to come from inside the individual concerned. It cannot be dropped into them like a blood transfusion, or wrapped around them like a bandage.

'John seemed to have a character change after his biopsy. He has such an enquiring mind usually, but he appeared to have switched his brain off – he just lay there like putty in the doctor's hands. I tried to get him to read some books I'd got – talk about how he felt and how he wanted to cope with things, but he wouldn't. In the end we had an argument – right there in the ward – in hissing whispers! Of course the chaplain had to choose that moment to come and visit John – and John didn't want to talk to him either – so the chaplain walked down to the lift with me instead. I poured it all out to him – how frightened and frustrated I was feeling because John didn't seem able to fight, and then he pointed out something that just hadn't occurred to me – that the best thing I could do was to surround John with a loving and supportive atmosphere and then trust him. John was still John, and becoming a cancer patient had not taken away his right to decide for himself. He reckoned this is how God treats us. Having made us beings with free will, he allows us to make our own decisions. When he sees those decisions are not really in our best interests, he doesn't "throw a switch" turning us into robots and taking away our freedom.

'I was afraid that if I took a step back from the situation it would look as if I didn't care, but the chaplain disagreed. He said that cutting back on my input of ideas and suggestions, and trusting John to make the right decision was not opting out, but actually being positively supportive. I needed to say, in attitude, if not in as many words, "I believe in you and your ability to make the best decisions for you. I'm here and I won't leave you; when you reach the point of needing help, I'll do all I can, if you let me know what you want."

'It was very hard for a "doer" like me to accept that he was right, and that there was nothing I *could* do to take John's pain and illness away from him… I had to realize that it was first and foremost *his* experience and *his* responsibility. I could bear it *with* him to a limited extent, but I could not bear it *for* him.'

And, of course, that is true for all of us. Whether patients want to take a passive or active role in their illness – or do the one thing today and the other thing tomorrow, as often happens – we can be involved only as supporters; we are not required to make a takeover bid.

Decision-making
Patients should not have to make snap decisions which have far-reaching results.

It is tough being in hospital for a number of reasons, not least on the decision-making front. Whether patients immediately accept the ward routine, or secretly think they could tell Sister a thing or two about people management, there usually comes a time when they begin to settle down. They come to terms with being told what to do for the majority of their waking hours, and then, perhaps after days of deciding nothing more demanding than what they will have to eat, the doctor comes along with the treatment plan. The patient is then likely to be faced with some life-changing choices, and is often expected to make an immediate decision.

'I seemed to spend days sitting around, waiting for tests to be done and the results to come back. Then all of a sudden the diagnosis was made, and I was told that I needed major surgery and I needed it straight away. It was urgent, they said, implying that if I didn't have it done immediately I'd be dead and done with. Faced with that, I panicked, said yes and signed the consent form. But I wasn't really convinced that I was doing the right thing, and I think that I would have coped with the after effects much better if I had stopped, thought it through, realized what the implications were and perhaps had a second opinion.'

The long-term outlook for this particular person was not really altered by the decision he made in haste, but that is not always the case. And this is where the first team supporters can have a helpful part to play. We can go over the implications of the treatment with the patient, clarify any uncertain areas by asking the doctor questions that the patient might have forgotten or felt unable to raise, and just act as a sounding board until they have talked it through to their satisfaction.

These are some of the questions that might usefully be asked at this point, in addition to those suggested earlier:

o What exactly is the treatment package that is being suggested? Is it surgery alone, or surgery plus radiotherapy or chemotherapy?

o Why is this particular treatment plan being advised? Are there any alternatives?

o How is the patient likely to feel afterwards – physically, emotionally and psychologically?

o What expert/lay assistance is available to help cope with these emotional and psychological needs?

o What are the side effects of the treatment likely to be?

o Where can we find more information if we want it?

o If the patient is treated as an outpatient (i.e. for radiotherapy or chemotherapy), what can we do at home to help in areas of diet, skin care, etc?

It is not being unduly fussy to look ahead like this. Forewarned is certainly forearmed in the treatment of cancer, as in anything else. And if satisfactory answers are not forthcoming, it is perfectly in order to ask for a second opinion. It is not considered to be a slur on the present doctor's abilities, and if it is difficult to approach the hospital doctor, your local doctor will arrange it if asked.

Fear and anxiety
One of the biggest fears that most of us have about cancer is that it will be very painful. In the event, it is not the physical pain that the majority find the hardest thing to grapple with in the first weeks after the disease is diagnosed, but the anxiety and uncertainty. If these feelings are bottled up, they can give rise to very real emotional suffering, and trigger off physical pain as well.

'I was aware of a growing inner sadness mingled with the recurrent fear. I longed somehow to express it and perhaps find an escape through crying, yet tears would give the lie to my careful cover-up and once I started crying it might be hard to stop. No, I must not let myself cry, I resolved, but maybe I could talk to someone…

'I realized that the "someone" would need to be outside my situation in order to be entirely objective. I missed Mary, the student nurse who had been such a friend. But Mary had gone, and I knew the doctors on our ward were far too busy for a long, somewhat complex offloading. How about the rest of the nursing staff? Somehow, for all their kindness, they seemed strangely unapproachable. Their work was done carefully and well, they anticipated and met requirements, but everything was kept very much to a practical level. The day-to-day programme didn't allow a slot for sitting and talking about deeper needs.'

Elaine is not alone in feeling too inhibited to share her feelings with others because they seem too busy, too detached (or not detached enough). In a study of patients who underwent surgery for breast cancer, seventy-eight per cent of the women questioned felt very anxious, but did not confide in anyone before surgery. In the first ten days after the operation forty-five per cent of them did share their worries, but more than half did not.

All sorts of reasons are given for not admitting how they felt.

'I didn't like to bother the staff. They've got so much to do, and no one likes a moaner.'

'I felt that I was lucky to have such a good prognosis, and it seemed almost wicked to complain about losing my breast if it was going to save my life. I kept looking round the ward and telling myself I should be grateful for what I'd got – but the misery kept coming back.'

'The nurses didn't seem to notice when I looked worried. I think they shut their eyes to it, really, because they didn't know what to say. Just talked about how well I was getting on and what they had done on their off-duty.'

'I was afraid they would stuff me full of tranquillizers if I admitted feeling depressed.'

'I felt that I couldn't worry my husband. He had got enough to do, coping at home, looking after the kids and getting to work on time. He was worn out with it all.'

First team supporters can do a lot to help in this situation, but that last comment does sum it up for some patients. They feel afraid of adding to the burdens that those they love are carrying, and try to spare them any further anxiety by pretending all is well. If this happens, someone who is a little less involved emotionally can often be very helpful. This may be one of the hospital personnel, such as the medical social worker, the chaplain or a specially trained nurse whose job it is to help those who have to adjust to mastectomies or colostomies. On the other hand, a sympathetic friend, or the minister of the patient's church, may be able to provide a very satisfactory listening ear.

These confidences cannot be dragged out of someone who is ill, but an opportunity often needs to be provided for them to be shared. The key seems to be to pick up the verbal clues that may be tossed out, seemingly quite casually, and handle them in the right way. For instance, the patient might say, 'I don't fancy the thought of an operation,' and we can easily respond by saying, 'Oh, they've got marvellous doctors here and they're doing your operation every day. There's no need to worry.' This will probably bring the patient's efforts to share their feelings to an abrupt end. However, if we say something like, 'What is it about the operation that you dread the most?' an opportunity is given to open up a little more.

Even a comment about what is going on physically can give an indication of how the person is feeling underneath. 'I've got a lot of pain today' can prompt a safe comment like, 'Well, you're bound to be sore after an operation' or, 'But you're looking so well!' or, 'Have you had any tablets lately?' What the patient may want to hear is, 'Have you any idea what is causing it?'

Having said all this, it does not mean that we have to look for hidden meanings in every innocent remark. Far from it. But as most of us are likely to give the 'safe' reply, almost without thinking, it is necessary to learn to be more sensitive. If the patient feels they cannot communicate in the way they really need to with those caring for them, their confidence will be eroded, they may well feel isolated and find it harder to cooperate with the treatment plan. This, in its turn, will undermine their recovery. So it will do no harm to think more carefully about when to be silent, when to speak, and what to say when you do – and it may do a great deal of good.

Help for supporters

'I just can't understand the way I felt when John was in hospital. One moment I was so thankful that someone else was taking the responsibility for his care – and then the next moment I was angry because they weren't giving him as much time and attention as I thought he should have. I criticized the way he had to wait for his medicine at times – and then felt really afraid that I would never cope with remembering all the different things he needed. And when he laughed and joked with the nurses I felt left out... a bit jealous, I suppose... it was as if I was on an emotional roller coaster that gave you a very bumpy ride!'

Jenny thought that her reactions were very odd, but she was only experiencing the hotchpotch of feelings that most of us have to cope with to some degree. There is a great potential for emotional tension when we see someone we love being admitted to hospital feeling ill, frightened and vulnerable. Our instinctive reaction is to protect them. And, since we cannot protect them from the cancer itself, we look around to see who or what else they need protecting from. Complaints about the shortcomings of the hospital system may stem from our own feeling of inadequacy because we cannot deal with the needs of 'our' patient as competently as the nurses do. We may then feel guilty for being so ungrateful.

It is very natural to feel this way, but it does not create the positive and cooperative atmosphere that is needed to help the patient most, and so it needs to be dealt with. The patient is *not* usually the best person onto whom to unload all these problems, especially as some of the negative feelings may directly concern them.

In our considerations so far I have assumed that the family relationship is close and happy, and that the patient's full recovery is the top priority for all concerned. But this is not always the case. Sometimes a partnership or other relationship is under considerable strain, and the news that one of those involved is seriously ill can arouse great feelings of guilt in the one who is well. This is either because the healthy partner feels that they have helped to bring about the illness in some way by their behaviour, or because they have a sense of relief when they realize that this illness could resolve the conflict by the death of one of the causes of it.

In all these delicate situations, we too need a 'listening ear' from someone who is outside of the problem. The same sources of professional help which are available to patients from within the hospital are usually there for the rest of the family too. Outside, the Samaritans will be happy to listen – they are *not* just concerned with potential suicides. So too will the minister of our local church, whether or not we attend regularly. Many doctors will also be glad to offer help. And if they feel they do not have enough time or expertise to see the needs properly met, they may well be able to recommend someone else who will. And, of course, we must not forget the one above all who has unlimited time and unlimited resources. Not only can God deal with our guilt by forgiving us: he can also enable us to forgive ourselves. So we should not feel too embarrassed or ashamed to admit our needs, or to make use of the help that is available if we are willing to ask for it.

8 Coping with the treatment

We have already had a brief look at the forms of routine medical treatment available to the cancer patient, and for those who want to explore the details, there is information available (see the book list on page 186). However, certain types of cancer treatment can face the patient and his or her family with wider problems than the obvious and immediate physical ones, and it is important to recognize them. We will take a look at these, but obviously each type of cancer brings its own specially sensitive areas. So at this point, be selective: read what applies to your own situation and ignore the rest.

Surgery

Any surgery equals loss. I have always thought that if I had cancer I would be so anxious to get rid of it that I would not mind what part of me had to be cut off or cut out in order to do so.

However, a recent blood test has made me see the whole thing in a new light. I have had plenty of blood tests in the past, and they have never bothered me at all. But as I watched the laboratory technician prepare to remove a syringeful from my arm that morning, I was struck with a sudden and inexplicable reluctance to allow her to continue.

'That is a part of me she's taking away,' I thought. 'She'll mess about with it and then throw it away.' And I did not like the thought of that at all.

This was quite a revelation to me. If I was (temporarily) so reluctant to part with a few millilitres of blood, which would be replaced by my own body within hours, I could now understand a little of what it must be like for people facing the loss of a far more important part of themselves. And yet we often tend to gloss over that aspect of surgery for cancer patients.

For breast cancer
Most women with cancer of the breast are faced with the prospect of an operation to remove all or part of the affected breast. There are three possible approaches to the surgery:

○ a **radical mastectomy**, which removes the whole of the breast tissue, the lymph glands under the arm and a major part of the underlying chest muscles. This is a very disfiguring operation, and since there is no statistical evidence to show that patients having such extensive surgery survive any better than those undergoing less radical techniques, it is often now replaced by

○ a **simple mastectomy**, which removes the breast and lymph glands but leaves the muscles in place. There is still a large scar and a loss of shape, but it is not quite so disfiguring. Some women who have a small lump in a medium-sized or larger breast are able to have

○ a **lumpectomy**, which removes the tumour and a small area of surrounding tissue but leaves the major part of the breast intact. A lumpectomy has to be followed by radiation therapy, to make sure that any cancer cells that are left behind are destroyed.

The surgeon will often remove lymph nodes from under the arm during the same operation, so that he can check whether the malignant cells have spread. If they have, the condition is described as 'node positive'. Further treatment will depend on whether there has been a spread of disease into the nodes.

Younger women (those who are before or at the menopause) who are 'node positive' may be offered chemotherapy with the hope that it will delay or prevent recurrence of their disease. The side effects of chemotherapy have to be balanced against the positive benefits, bearing in mind that only about fifty per cent of women will have a recurrence of their breast cancer within ten years anyway.

The growth of some tumours is influenced by hormones, and it is now possible to test the tissue taken from the tumour to see if it is hormone responsive. If it is, hormone treatment can be given if the cancer recurs.

From these facts, it is easy to see that a mastectomy patient has a great deal to contend with. In common with other cancer sufferers she may have worries about:

o whether all the cancer has been removed

o how far it had progressed

o whether it will recur

o what further treatment will involve.

In addition, she is likely to feel anxious about:

o her own attractiveness

o the reaction of her partner (if she has one) and the rest of her family and close friends

o the problems of having an artificial breast (a prothesis) – will it fit, will it show, will it look natural?

o the problems of choosing suitable clothes and trying them on in this era of communal changing rooms.

Good pre-operative counselling and reassurance about the help which will be available to her makes a great difference to the mastectomy patient but, even so, many women experience some degree of depression during the first year after the operation. About ten per cent find that they have a marked reduction in their interest in sex; a far greater number find it difficult to look at their scar themselves or allow their partner to do so, and the majority seem reluctant to buy new clothes for a while.

'If you have had a mastectomy you need constant, and I *mean* constant, reassurance that you are still needed as a woman. Losing my breast meant for me a devastating attack on my femininity.'

'My personal life has suffered – my husband and I have survived, but only just at times. If only we had had more counselling *together* at the beginning, we would have been spared a lot of heartache.'

'I looked in the mirror and I didn't like what I saw. But then I thought, "I'd rather be alive and lopsided than dead." And that was that, really.'

The way that a woman copes with the situation seems to depend on a number of things. She feels most positive if:

o she is given a good outlook for the future by her doctor

o her own view of her physical attractiveness is not orientated towards the shape and size of her bust

o her husband or partner is able to offer very positive reassurance about her sex appeal and does not react negatively to her scar. *Genuine* assurance of love, and a refusal to allow her to withdraw from mixing socially, avoid love-making or conceal her scar from him goes a long way towards restoring a woman's shaken confidence.

A number of women are dissatisfied with their false breast, finding it too heavy, or that it slips out of their bra. Research shows that few of them actually mention the problem, and that is another area where we, as relatives, can help and encourage them to make use of the resources available. Many hospitals have a trained mastectomy nurse attached to the breast clinic who can be of tremendous assistance in practical ways as well as in emotional and sexual counselling. They will also be a useful source of information for those women who want to explore the possibility of breast reconstruction, either immediately or months or years later. There are several methods of rebuilding the breast, and although there is no hurry to decide, if the patient knows that she wants to consider this option before she has her mastectomy, it is helpful to discuss it with her surgeon pre-operatively as this may influence the way the initial surgery is carried out. Help is also available through organizations specializing in this problem (see the list of useful addresses on page 188) and local cancer support groups.

For cancer of the reproductive system

Some women feel a considerable degree of loss and distress if they have their womb (uterus) and/or ovaries removed. Again, there is the implied threat to their femininity – especially for those to whom childbearing is a crucial part of being a woman. This is particularly difficult for women who have no children and had hoped to have them, or those who feel that their family is not complete. They need very similar encouragement and support to the mastectomy patient, for their sense of loss, although less physically obvious, can go just as deep.

For prostate cancer

Men who have prostate cancer have a number of treatment options available to them, including surgery and radiation therapy. Both of these forms of treatment have the potential for serious and life-changing side effects, principally impotence (the inability to have an erection or father children) and incontinence (the inability to control their urine).

The possibility of the loss of an active sex life can be potentially devastating for both partners, and some men will even decline these forms of treatment because of the problems that might ensue.

'We had always enjoyed a good love life and the thought of it ending was unbearable. I was all set to refuse the operation, until my surgeon pointed out that I wouldn't be having any hot dates in the cemetery. I know that it was hard for my wife too, but she said that she would rather have me and perhaps no sex, than be without me, and we have compensated up to a point. But it was a tough choice, and a long time before I felt like a man again.'

This is a situation where both partners will need pre-operative counselling, as impotence can be helped in a number of ways.

The patient will also be shown how to do pelvic floor exercises by the physiotherapist, and reassured that although there will almost certainly be some loss of control first, most men have made the adjustment within the first year after treatment. But these very intimate problems do cause distress, and a similar degree of sensitivity and support is needed for a prostate cancer patient post treatment as for women who have had a mastectomy.

For head and neck cancer

People with tumours of the jaw, neck and face can be treated by surgical removal of the affected area and have a very good future outlook in terms of length of life. However, the operation itself can be very disfiguring and, if the larynx is affected, the patient will have the additional problem of learning to speak in a new way. Unless there is very active support from family and friends, sufferers from this form of cancer can become very withdrawn. A positive and encouraging attitude is vital, both before the operation and afterwards.

Before the operation it is the consultant's responsibility to explain to the patient and their family what is to be done, and what to expect afterwards. This is a time when denial can reassert itself, so that the full implications are not really absorbed. Once again we need to ask questions about anything that is not clear, and we need to encourage the patient to talk as freely as they are able to about the problems that lie ahead and how they will be faced. Readjustment can be made more difficult because people suffering from this kind of cancer are often in the older age group and may find it less easy to adapt.

If the speech is likely to be affected, the speech therapist will probably visit the patient before the operation so that he or she knows them and can reassure them that they are not going to be incommunicado for the rest of their life. After a laryngectomy (removal of the voice box), the patient can often be taught to speak using the oesophagus. This can sound quite natural and the speech therapist may arrange for another patient who has already learned to speak well in this way to visit the patient and demonstrate their skills. Of course, this is more encouraging than anything the medical team can say.

After the operation, there may be stiffness of the neck and shoulders which can be considerably helped by physiotherapy. The patient will have problems eating and drinking at first, and a liquidizer is a great help in making food edible. Many hospital social services departments can arrange for the patient to be supplied with a liquidizer for use at home if one is not already available.

The biggest hurdle of all is the need to accept a change in appearance, and it is here that family and friends can be of most use.

If we can accept the 'new look' and constantly assure the patient of our love and support – touch is all important in expressing this and helping the patient to realize that we are not withdrawing from them – self-acceptance will be much easier. Some hospitals arrange for patients to face the outside world very soon after surgery. As soon as they are well enough, they are encouraged to dress and go out to the shops with a relative or perhaps a nurse. This may seem cruel, but like any other difficult undertaking, the sooner it is faced, the easier it is to cope with in the long run. However, we must never trivialize the problems or expect constant cheerfulness and courage (from ourselves or the patient). Adaptation and acceptance are not automatic: they are processes that take time and cannot be hurried.

For bowel and bladder cancer

When someone is suffering from a tumour in the bowel or urinary tract (and certain other diseases), it is sometimes necessary to make a new route for discharging the body's waste products. This is either because the cancer is blocking the normal route, or because, in removing the tumour, the intestine has been so damaged that it can no longer function properly. The new pathway is created in an operation called an *ostomy*, and the opening on to the body's surface is called a *stoma*. The *colostomy* is an opening from any part of the large bowel or colon. An *ileostomy* is made using the ileum, which is the part of the small intestine farthest from the stomach. Both of these stomas discharge stools into a bag attached to it. An ileal conduit bypasses the bladder and allows urine to be drained through a segment of the ileum. The rest of the bowel works normally after this operation.

We have only to think how embarrassed we feel when we have a rumbling stomach or wind in a crowded room (or even with two or three other people) to have an inkling of the problems that face a stoma patient.

Doctors insist that it is perfectly possible to resume a normal life in every way after such an operation. This may be so, but it is not a very easy task to convince the patient of that in the early days after surgery. If mastectomy patients feel threatened by diminution of their sexual identity and attractiveness, people with a stoma have to face the fact that one of the most private parts of their bodily system is no longer under their voluntary control. Since we are conditioned to think of lack of control of bowels and bladder as something belonging to babyhood, it is not hard to understand the sense of actual and psychological loss that is involved.

It is very important that anyone who is facing this operation has extensive preparation beforehand. Many surgeons explain where the opening will be and mark it on the patient's stomach, having seen them standing up and lying down. This is because it is essential for the patient to be able to see their stoma in order to deal with it properly. Some hospitals have a stoma clinic, attended by specially trained nurses and other patients who are coping with their appliance successfully. A visit there before the operation is invaluable for the patient and relatives. Their questions can be answered and their fears dispelled – at least in part.

What is it that a stoma patient fears, apart from loss of control over their bodily functions?

They fear that the stoma bag may not work efficiently and that there could be leakage, offensive smells and noises, which would be both embarrassing for them and unpleasant for others.

This fear of social contact is heightened by the thought of physical intimacy with their husband or wife. If a mastectomy patient is afraid that her lopsided appearance when undressed will make her sexually unattractive, it is easy to see that the thought of an appliance on your stomach, into which potentially offensive material might discharge itself, is equally unattractive. There is also the fear that close physical contact may harm the colostomy or lead to spillage. Some men also have the problem that nerves are damaged during the operation, resulting in total impotence or some reduction in their ability to enjoy love-making.

There is also fear of the actual management of the colostomy, what they will be able to eat and drink and how this will affect their social and working life.

Given all these very real fears, it is not surprising that after a stoma operation many people suffer from:

o depression – of varying degrees of severity

o anxiety about keeping clean – some patients become obsessed with the need to wash the area around the colostomy repeatedly o sexual problems

o reduction in their social activities. In a study carried out in 1976 as many as eighteen per cent of people had refused to go on holiday or spend even a night away from home because of anxiety about dealing with their colostomies and disposing of their colostomy bags in strange surroundings.

In the light of all this, it is obvious that both patient and relatives will face a changed lifestyle. Once again, the most important things we can offer are constant reassurance, both physically and verbally; practical help in things like experimenting to find the best diet; and providing privacy and encouragement while the patient gets used to handling the appliance.

There are self-help groups and organizations which give advice and personal support (see the list of useful addresses on page 188). Home and hospital visiting is an important part of their work and all speak from personal experience.

Most of all, we need to keep the goal of a return to normal living prominently in our sights. We may not make it all the way. We may have to accept that, for our family, normality from now on will be different. But it is amazing what can be achieved in this, as in every other area of adjustment after surgery, if we accentuate the positive, eliminate the negative, and appreciate every step accomplished as a bonus to be celebrated.

Radiation therapy

Radiation in any form tends to have a very bad press these days, and the knowledge that part of their body is deliberately being exposed to concentrated doses of X-rays generates quite a large degree of anxiety in most people. The fact that it is intended for your good does not relieve that anxiety overmuch, particularly when you are faced with a huge machine that whirrs and hums, and a radiographer who disappears into another room while it is working, leaving you apparently at its mercy. Add to this the fact that most people who are having radiotherapy are likely to be either recovering from recent surgery, or battling with a recurrence of their disease, and it is easy to see why radiation treatment often has rather a depressing effect.

Some patients have their radiotherapy treatment as inpatients, either because they live a long way from the hospital, or because they are not well enough to make even a short journey on a regular basis. But many are able to be at home and attend the hospital four or five times a week for two to four weeks. Each patient's treatment is individually planned, so the frequency of visits may vary, but if they are treated as outpatients, those of us looking after them at home will need to be well informed about what is going on, so that we can offer the best possible care.

These are some of the questions that it may be useful to ask the doctor (radiotherapist) before radiotherapy begins.

o How long will the treatment go on for?

o How long will each individual session take?

o Will it be done as an inpatient or an outpatient?

o What is the treatment expected to achieve?

o What side effects should we expect?

o Will these be short term (like tiredness or sickness) or long term (as with a decrease in fertility)?

o What can we do to care for the patient's general well-being, their skin, their diet?

o Are there any special precautions that need to be taken?

o Can the patient get him or herself to and from hospital or will they need help?

What happens during treatment?
The first visit to the radiotherapy department is usually for a planning session. The area to be treated is marked on the patient's body with a purple dye – which must not be washed off during the period of treatment – or small dots. The radiotherapist plans the treatment and works out the dose of radiation needed with a radiation physicist. This dose is then divided into small parts or 'fractions' and given as individual treatments.

The treatment is given by a radiographer, who has been specially trained to give radiotherapy in addition to his or her basic training in taking diagnostic X-rays. They will place the patient in the correct position, shield any parts of the body that need protecting from the radiation, and position the machine. They will not stay in the same room as the patient during treatment, but can see them through a thickened glass window or TV screen, and speak to them over a loudspeaker system. They will watch the patient right through the period of treatment, which is usually only a few minutes.

What are the problems to look out for?

o Anxiety and depression are common. We have already seen that the patient may feel anxious because of the frightening undertones associated with the very word radiation. They already have to cope with the anxiety associated with the fact that they have cancer, so there is a tendency to worry about problems produced by the treatment itself – which can seem very much like the symptoms of the original cancer. When this happens, patients tend to forget (unless reminded) that they have been warned about side effects, and fear that the cancer is recurring, or getting worse, and not responding to treatment.

o Tiredness is the most common side effect of radiotherapy and builds up as the treatment progresses, often reaching a peak up to six weeks after the course of therapy is completed. It is useful to realize this because tiredness tends to increase anxiety and depression, and also because it is easy to imagine that the patient is making a fuss unnecessarily if they are still complaining of feeling exhausted for quite a while after all the obvious reasons for it have gone.

o Loss of appetite and nausea. Some people are feeling sick and unlike eating long before their radiation treatment begins. If they are depressed, it obviously all seems worse. If the stomach is being irradiated this will be likely to provide digestive upsets. Radiotherapy to the head and neck can result in a dry and sore mouth, sore throat and alterations in taste. It may cause either complete loss of taste or make some foods, previously enjoyed, taste unpleasant. Needless to say, all this makes food seem very unattractive, and it is quite a test of ingenuity to make it enjoyable. These are some of the ways that we can help.

Forget about high fibre and raw foods if the patient has diarrhoea, or is finding it hard to chew. A soft high protein diet with plenty of fluid is needed. Sometimes it is helpful to liquidize the meal (item by item, not in a mass so that it looks like baby food). Avoid fried or fatty food.

Serve food in small amounts and frequently. Some people prefer to eat quietly by themselves, because the smell of the family's meal can increase their nausea.

Presentation is important. Small plates, and food attractively arranged, stimulate the appetite. So does a tart-tasting fruit juice or a glass of sherry before the meal. Some people cope better with warm rather than hot food.

Sucking ice cubes flavoured with fruit juice, or lemon drops or other acid sweets, helps to stimulate the flow of saliva.

It is important that patients eat and maintain body weight. But it is also important that eating does not become a battleground between patients and those caring for them. A relaxed approach and a willingness to experiment with different foods can make all the difference, just as it does in the case of small children who have eating problems. And we must not take it personally when our lovingly prepared meals are put on one side after two or three mouthfuls. It is easy to feel that *we* are being rejected as well as the food, but that is not really the case, and it is counterproductive to let it spoil our day.

If it is possible to establish a good diet with the patient so that they are well-nourished before treatment starts, it is a great help in reducing side effects. It is not necessary to eat more in order to do this, if we use our dietary know-how to add extra protein and calories to a light diet. For instance:

~egg beaten up in milk with a dash of vanilla essence tastes like liquid ice cream

~jellies can be made with milk, and so can soup

~eggs can be added to mashed potato, and so can grated cheese

~yoghurt can be added to sauces and puréed with fruit

~extra butter and cheese can raise the calorie content, but be careful of overdoing the fat content of the meal

~protein supplements (e.g. Complan, Build Up) can be made into nourishing drinks, and some people like them. Glucose drinks are also beneficial. Calorie supplements can be added to both sweet and savoury foods. All of these can be bought at most chemists. Your doctor may also prescribe feeds which can be made up to suit the patient's individual needs.

o Skin irritation. The skin over the area can become sore during radiation therapy. A mild redness is not important and will disappear after treatment is complete. Calamine lotion is soothing for any itchiness which develops, but check with the radiotherapist before using it.

The skin can be washed with warm water, but no soap should be used on the general treatment area and especially on the planning marks.

Ointments, perfume, cosmetics and hot water bottles should also be kept away from treated skin during treatment and for at least ten days afterwards. Any shaving should be done with an electric razor if the face is being treated.

Occasionally the skin breaks down and becomes red and weepy. If this happens the radiotherapist or radiographer should be told. Gentian violet is often used to dry the affected area, but sometimes a hydro-cortisone cream may be needed. Loose, soft clothing, with no tight straps or collars, will help to prevent rubbing and subsequent soreness.

o Hair loss can occur when the head is treated, but it is always temporary. The hair grows back, although it may not be the same colour or texture, when the treatment is completed. Nevertheless, it is very upsetting for the person concerned and should not be taken lightly. It is possible for wigs to be supplied on the National Health Service, and these can be chosen before the hair loss happens, which makes the patient feel more secure and cared for. Some people do not like wigs, though, and prefer to make do with hats and scarves.

o It is important that teeth are in a good condition before treatment begins, if the radiotherapy is to involve the mouth. If possible, the patient should have a dental check-up and any treatment that is needed before radiation therapy is given. The dentist should be told the situation. Teeth need to be cleaned frequently – up to four times a day – with a soft brush, and the mouth well rinsed. A home-made mouth wash consisting of two pints of warm water in which one teaspoon of salt and one teaspoon of baking soda have been dissolved is better than commercially-produced rinses, which often contain alcohol. Always tell the dentist if radiotherapy has been given to the face or jaw, for at least the first year after treatment.

Chemotherapy

Anti-cancer drug therapy is an area of cancer treatment which is developing and expanding all the time. Patients who are treated by this method have to face the fact that it causes more side effects than the other forms of cancer therapy, and so the effectiveness of the treatment has to be weighed against these possible unpleasant side effects. Some of the more unusual tumours can actually be cured by anti-cancer drugs. In this situation it is obviously worth putting up with a great deal during the treatment in order to be free of the disease.

Other cancers cannot be cured, but drug therapy is useful to relieve symptoms and prolong life.

Obviously the doctor would want to be able to offer a considerable improvement of symptoms, or a substantially increased life expectancy, before asking the patient to embark on a long course of regular inpatient treatments, frequent visits to monitor drugs taken at home, and side effects which might range in severity from mildly inconvenient to downright unpleasant.

So it is very important to discuss the treatment fully before it begins. Some of the questions to ask would be:

o What will the drug therapy be likely to achieve – a cure, or relief of symptoms?

o Why is it the best form of treatment for the patient now?

o How long would it continue?

o How long would each session of treatment last?

o How are the drugs given?

o Will it be necessary to go into hospital for treatment, or can it be given on an outpatient basis?

o What are the immediate/long-term side effects?

o Will it affect fertility permanently or temporarily (and can sperm or ova be banked), and does it matter if the patient becomes pregnant during treatment?

o If the patient develops any of these side effects, does anyone need to be told?

o If so, how do we get in touch with them and how urgent is it?

If chemotherapy has been decided upon, it is important to encourage the patient to have a positive approach. Not everyone has severe side effects and what happens does seem to depend, to a degree, on the patient's own attitude.

'My husband was very resistant to the idea of chemotherapy. He was doing everything to rid his body of toxins by diet, visualization and mental attitude. He was confronted with the prospect of a treatment which he was told would save his life, and if he didn't have it he would die. He saw this treatment as being fed with more toxins.

'He struggled with that dilemma, which could be seen as, "If I have it I'll die, and if I don't have it I'll die." In the end he saw that he could experience it another way and he chose to have the treatment and for it to work. He sat up all night with someone who was starting his course, watched his reactions and saw that he himself could choose to experience it differently. He managed to create around him a very powerful atmosphere of patience and calm. We both found a lot of comfort from the "Just for today" card published by Alcoholics Anonymous. It starts:

"Just for today I will try to live through this day only and not tackle my whole life problem at once. I can do something for twelve hours that would appal me if I felt I had to keep it up for a lifetime."

'His response to the treatment was good and he had less intensive side effects than many. He had very little nausea and was able to eat normally, putting on weight, which is the opposite to most people's experience.'

This patient had weighed up all the pros and cons and had come to an informed and deliberate decision. That factor is a very important one. We often tend to forget that no one can be forced to have any form of treatment against their will. A cancer patient is still someone with the right to choose. Having chosen to have chemotherapy, with full knowledge of what the side effects may be, the patient will still need support in coping with them. Different drugs cause different problems, but, in general terms, what is the worst that we may have to face?

o Tiredness, sickness and loss of appetite. These reactions are similar to those caused by radiotherapy and should be handled in much the same way. Vomiting can be a very troublesome reaction to some drugs. In addition to observing the simple guidelines of eating light meals frequently and avoiding fried and fatty foods, tablets and injections can be given to control the sickness.

Very occasionally the vomiting can be so traumatic that the patient finds it almost impossible to cooperate with the treatment. But there is help at hand, even for this.

Tim Dean had the unpleasant experience, common to many chemotherapy patients, of feeling relatively well between his drug therapy sessions, and so it seemed that he was going into hospital to be made to feel extremely ill, rather than to be made better. His drugs were given by injection and in tablet form and always made him violently sick. After three sessions Tim found himself totally unable to face swallowing the pills and, when he did try to do so, he simply vomited them up almost immediately. He had developed a pill phobia. Even the sight of a pill on the cinema screen made him feel ill. It was essential that he continued with the treatment, because Tim's form of cancer, Hodgkin's disease, is curable by chemotherapy. Without it he would die.

Help came to him in the shape of a clinical psychologist. She helped Tim to overcome his aversion to tablets by teaching him to relax and measure his level of relaxation using a bio-feedback machine. This is a simple device which is strapped to the hand. It measures the degree of tension the patient is feeling by the amount of sweating that is taking place. As Tim learned to relax, the machine recorded the fact by giving off a gentle bleep instead of a high-pitched whine. Once he was relaxed he took pill-shaped sweets. When he could cope with those without fear, he was able, with a lot of support and encouragement, to return to his drug treatment.

o A sore mouth is another side effect shared with radiotherapy. Good mouth care – regular brushing of teeth and mouth washes; avoidance of salty and spicy foods which may give a burning sensation, and eating soft food (liquidized if necessary), are all easy steps to take that will help the situation.

   If the soreness becomes severe, or white patches develop in the mouth, the doctor should be consulted, as this needs treating with a special mouth wash.

o Hair loss. Chemotherapy affects the whole body, so hair loss does not depend on whether the patient's head is being treated (as in radiotherapy) but on whether the drugs being used are the types which attack the cells in the hair follicles. If they are, the same management is employed – a wig for those who want one, and plenty of reassurance that the situation is only temporary. It is important to realize, though, that 'temporary' may seem quite a long while to the patient, if the treatment goes on over a period of months. Most of us are extremely sensitive about our appearance.

'Betsy is normally full of fun, able to take a joke better than most people I know. One morning I propped her new wig jauntily on my head and began clowning for Suzanne and Marybeth. It was a painful miscalculation. Betsy was excruciatingly sensitive to our daughters' reaction to having "a mother who's going bald". The wig was an ever-present reminder of her loss. And without ever meaning to, I had trampled across the line into an area where teasing was no longer funny but hurtful.'

o Skin irritation. Allergic skin rashes may develop during treatment and can be treated by tablets. If a combination of drugs is being taken, the doctor will usually try to find out which one is causing the trouble.

Some drugs can damage the skin and surrounding tissues if they leak from the vein while being injected. This is not a time for the patient to be brave. If there is pain during an injection into the vein, the doctor or nurse should be told, as the leaked drug can cause a sore or ulcer which is very difficult to heal.

o Bone marrow damage. The three types of cell that circulate in the blood are manufactured in the bone marrow. Because it is an area of rapid cell division, the chemotherapy drugs are likely to damage these blood cells as well as the cancer cells in other parts of the body.

~The *red cells* carry oxygen round the body. Damage to them results in anaemia, and patients may feel tired and irritable, dizzy, short of breath and cold.

~The *white cells* fight infection. If the white cell count is low, people catch infectious diseases very easily.

~The *platelets* are the clotting cells in the blood which make sure we don't bleed to death if we cut ourselves. Lack of platelets results in uncontrolled bleeding.

If these cells are damaged they will replace themselves quite quickly, but during chemotherapy patients will have blood tests before treatment is given, to make sure the bone marrow has done its job. If it has not, a transfusion may be necessary before treatment continues.

To help protect themselves during the entire period of chemotherapy, patients should:

~avoid crowded places and people with infectious diseases

~be careful not to cut or scratch the skin when doing dirty jobs

~avoid medicines containing aspirin if the blood platelet count is low, because aspirin damages platelets at the best of times

~watch out for unexplained bruises, bleeding from the nose or gums, or blood in the urine.

If any of the following symptoms occurs, the doctor should be contacted promptly:

~a high temperature, cough or feeling very hot, cold and/or shivering

~unexplained bruising or bleeding that will not stop

~burning pain when passing urine or blood in the urine

~any of the symptoms of anaemia

~diarrhoea that lasts for more than forty-eight hours

~lack of coordination or loss of balance

~severe constipation

~pins and needles affecting the whole hand or foot and difficulty in holding small objects

~deafness

The last four problems can be caused by certain drugs that affect the central nervous system, and need immediate attention.

o Mood changes. Some drugs in themselves cause an alteration in the patient's mental and emotional well-being. In addition, there is the emotional strain of the disease itself and of prolonged and unpleasant treatment.

'After my fourth monthly session of drug therapy I just fell into a pit of despair. The whole world seemed completely black. I couldn't remember it ever being any different in the past and I couldn't believe that it would ever be any different in the future. It was a totally overwhelming experience. I had no wish to get out of bed – what was there to get up for? The only person who got through to me at all was my sister. She just sat and held my hand and kept repeating a funny little phrase, "It came to pass..." She reminded me over and over again that it was the drugs that were making me feel so ghastly, that it had come and it would pass, and that God *was* there in the shadows. It did pass eventually and I was so thankful that she kept on reassuring me, even though I didn't respond at the time. I couldn't put it into words, but

I thought that I was going mad. I hung on to the fact that it was the drugs, not me, when I had to face the next lot of treatment, and it was never as bad again.'

Strictly practical
We have already given considerable thought to the emotional and physical care a cancer patient needs during treatment. However, there are a few other practical points which may seem obvious but are things which a number of cancer patients wished others had borne in mind.

o Visitors do not have to talk a lot. In fact, if the patient is feeling tired or ill, it is often better if they do not. Just being there is reassuring and touch is so important – a hug, a kiss, a hand held makes them feel less like a leper. Cancer is not catching.

o It is lovely to keep in touch with the family, but not all at once. If visiting can be staggered it is much more enjoyable and less tiring for the patient. A certain amount of tactful organization might be needed to ensure that this happens.

o People hate to visit a hospital empty-handed, but some gifts are more appropriate than others:

~Magazines are often easier to hold and concentrate on than books and can be passed on to other patients.

~A small photo album filled with pictures of family and special happy occasions can be both a talking point and a mood lifter.

~Cassettes, CDs or a personal stereo require less effort than reading.

~A pot plant is a symbol of life... cut flowers die.

~Perfumed toiletries can be lovely, but can also be a cause of nausea for some people.

~Lip salve for dry lips and boiled sweets to suck can help with a dry mouth, but beware of bringing too much food. If your appetite is limited, a basket of fruit can seem overwhelming. A small bowl of cherries or strawberries, on the other hand, can tempt a jaded palate. One man's best present in the food line was a tin of his favourite chicken soup – which was not an item that would occur to most people!

o It is difficult to concentrate in the hustle and bustle of a busy ward. Patients who at home would normally read their Bible and pray often find it hard to do in hospital.

Amy was glad when people wrote out Bible verses in full for her on their get well cards, instead of just putting the reference. She was able to enjoy their comfort without having to make the effort to look them up.

Gary and his wife usually prayed together each evening and he was glad when she suggested, a little nervously, that she should pray for them both for a moment before she went home. The first night they drew the curtain slightly around the bed, but after that they lost their embarrassment. And Gary was both touched and heartened to find that, far from mocking him, the patient in the next bed asked if they would pray for him too.

9 Working together

When we are watching someone whom we love struggling to cope with the after effects of surgery or the side effects of radiation or chemotherapy, it is very natural to feel that our own needs are totally unimportant in comparison with theirs. But this is a mistake.

Our own needs
If we are going to be able to give our physical and emotional energy as freely as we would wish to do, our own resources have to be replenished. The two biggest areas of stress and strain seem to be keeping things going fairly normally at home and coping with constant hospital visiting. These are some of the solutions that other people have worked out.

'When people asked how they could help, I could never think of anything on the spur of the moment, and anyway I didn't really like to take advantage of their kindness. Then one day I had ironing piled so high I couldn't lift the basket and my next-door neighbour came in. She saw the pile of shirts and just picked up the basket without a word and took it home. She returned the shirts while I was at the hospital that evening – all beautifully ironed. After that it was easier to accept help, and I started keeping a little list of odd jobs that needed doing. When friends asked what they could do I was ready with a choice – which gave some of them quite a shock!'

'One of the worst things about Mike being in hospital was that the phone just didn't stop ringing from the time I got home from evening visiting until I went to bed. It was so exhausting repeating the same things over and over again. In the end Mike's brother offered to take that over. I rang him as soon as I got in (if he hadn't visited for a day or two) with up to date news, and gave his number to everyone who was likely to phone. A few people still came straight to me, but it was much easier to cope with.'

'We seemed to get so little time alone. I appreciated the fact our friends wanted to visit, but I wanted my husband to myself. It was hard to pluck up the courage to ask them not to come on a Monday night, but, when I did, it took a lot of the tension out of the situation and no one was obviously offended.'

'Sister took me on one side one evening. She said that I looked worn out, and she was right. I had been visiting afternoon and evening for three weeks and I never seemed to stop running. She told me quite firmly that I should take three afternoons off a week and do something for myself – not use the time to catch up on housework. When I went to the hairdresser's instead of the hospital I felt really guilty, but I felt so much better afterwards, and my father seemed to be rather more cheered up by a well-groomed visitor than a zombie!'

Children also suffer when their parents are ill or preoccupied with hospital visiting and, although they may not say very much, their behaviour often speaks volumes. It is important to explain to them as much of the situation as they are able to understand and to include them in visiting and helping in small ways, so that they do not feel isolated. It is also wise to tell their teachers what is happening at home, so that they are not put under pressure at school.

The doctor's point of view
Doctors, patients and relatives all have expectations about one another's behaviour and ability to meet the demands of an illness such as cancer. Whether or not those expectations are fulfilled will determine whether the group can work together as a team, or whether they will all be circling around each other, getting nowhere.

What should we be able to expect from the doctor?
We should expect full and frank discussion – but we should be prepared to ask questions and not expect the doctor to be a mind reader.

The doctor will take the responsibility for recommending the best course of treatment in his or her view, and be open-minded enough to obtain a second opinion for us if required. However, the final decision must ultimately rest with the patient.

The doctor will see the patient as a person, not merely a disease, and take their social, emotional and psychological needs into account when making decisions.

The doctor will be honest. He or she may not be able to say exactly what any one individual's reaction to treatment will be, but they can say what usually happens, and whether we can expect this disease to follow the normal pattern.

The doctor will be emotionally supportive, and even if they reach the end of active treatment options, they will remain encouraging and hopeful. They will not allow the patient to feel that he or she has been abandoned. The doctor will aim to manage the needs of the patient rather than merely treat the disease.

Having listed these sterling qualities which most doctors would *want* to offer, we must realize that they are human beings and will fail at times. One of the most important things to grasp is that in the past medical students have been taught that successful treatment in *their* terms is a matter of applying the appropriate techniques for the removal of the disease. If these techniques do not work, or they run out of options to try, there is a real sense of failure. It seems that the disease has won. What happens with the *body* is seen as all-important. This approach goes back a long way. Even the ancient Greeks must have thought like this, because Plato wrote, 'For this is the greatest error of our day, that in treating the human body, physicians separate the soul from the body.'

This attitude is not as common now. More training schools are teaching their student doctors to look at the whole person, and not just the illness. But it will take time to work right through the system, and old habits die hard.

Because of this, doctors still tend to see death as the ultimate failure on their part, and many of them find it difficult to accept the human limitations on their profession. Add to this the fact that doctors are just as likely as the rest of the human race to fear death, unless they have some inner spiritual resources. (White coats can be used as a cover for negative emotions, but they do not make the wearer immune.) Grasp that and you can imagine what it might cost someone who felt both powerless and fearful to have to break the news of a terminal illness to their patient.

It is *never* easy. Most of us tend to avoid feelings of failure by withdrawing from the person or thing that makes us feel that way. This is why patients sometimes complain that they feel put to one side, that the doctor has lost interest in them when active treatment ceases.

What should the doctor be able to expect from us?
A willingness to listen and be guided, but also to take responsibility for our own decisions.

A realization that, however vital and desperate our particular cancer crisis is to us, we are only one of a number of families that they are responsible for.

An effort to listen to instructions and carry them out to the best of our ability, to ask if we do not understand, and to observe the prescribed times for appointments, telephone calls and visits, unless it is a real emergency.

Not to demand of them more than we would ask of ourselves in terms of time, patience, understanding and wisdom.

To realize that they may still be grappling with their own reactions to a disease like cancer, and that this may make them more negative and less supportive than we would like them to be. (If this is the case, we have two options: one is to work with them as far as possible whilst realizing that some of our support, at least, will have to come from elsewhere. The other is to change our doctor. But this should be a last resort rather than first reaction.)

Cancer is a disease that has to be fought on every level – by the body, the mind, the emotions and the spirit. That is a very tall order and can only be done with real success when all involved work together in loving cooperation. The following paraphrase of Paul's letter to the

Corinthians, chapter 13, written by Dr Ernesto Contreras, was intended for doctors, but I think that it has something to say to every member of the cancer-fighting force.

'Though I become a famous scientist or practising physician, and I display in my office many diplomas and degrees, and I am considered as an excellent teacher or convincing speaker, but have no love, I am just a sounding brass or a tinkling cymbal.

And though I have the gift of being an unusual clinician making the most difficult diagnoses; and understand all the mysteries of the human body; and feel sure I can treat any kind of diseases, even cancer; but have no love, I am nobody.

And though I invest all my money to build the best facilities, buy the best equipment, have the most prominent physicians for the sake of my patients; and I devote all my time for their care, even to the point of neglecting my own family or myself; but have not love, it profiteth me nothing.

Love is an excellent medicine, it is non-toxic; it does not depress the body defence, but enhances it.

It can be combined with all kinds of remedies, acting as a wonderful positive catalyst.

It relieves pain and maintains quality of life at its best level.

It is tolerated by anyone; never causes allergies or intolerance.

Common medicines come and go. What was considered good yesterday is useless now. What is considered good now will be worthless tomorrow. But love has passed all tests and will be effective always.

We now know things only partially, and most therapies are only experimental.

But when all things are understood we will recognize the value of love.

It is the only agent capable of creating good rapport between patients, relatives and doctors, so everybody will not act as children but as mature people.

Today many truths appear as blurred images to us as physicians, and we can't understand how the things of the spirit work to maintain life; but one day we will see all things very clearly.

And now remain three basic medications: faith, hope and love, but the greatest of these is love.'

PART TWO:
The intermediate stage

10 First days at home

During the battle against cancer, it is quite likely that someone will be admitted to hospital and come home again more than once. It may well be what the media people like to call an ongoing situation.

However, for the purpose of our thinking at this point, I am assuming that the patient is coming home after the first major session of treatment and that they are in complete remission. This means that the tumour has completely disappeared (or been completely removed) and that all the tests which previously showed an abnormality are now clear. (If the tumour has shrunk to less than half of its original size and has stayed that way for more than one month, the patient is said to be in partial remission.)

Doctors are very wary about pronouncing a patient cured of cancer. They will think of doing that only when a person has been in complete remission for a number of years. The exact length of time varies from tumour to tumour, but a rough guide is around five years. The risk of a recurrence of the disease is at its highest during the first year after treatment has been completed, and diminishes every year after that. So the patient has a long road to travel before they can confidently say that they are cured, and even if the outlook is good – and we are assuming for the moment that it is – we will all (patient and family alike) need a great deal of support and encouragement during the early days, as we aim to help:

o build as full a physical recovery as possible

o come to terms with the use of any appliance, or the sense of physical mutilation which may exist o pick up the threads of the patient's social and working life

o together discover the kind of lifestyle that will fit in with the circumstances in which we now find ourselves – working, not to get back to life as it was, necessarily, but to move on, to create a new normality.

'It will be all right when I get home'

When someone is in hospital, going home is often felt to be the potential solution to all their problems, from not being able to eat to having an allergic reaction to sticking plaster. Such high hopes are built up that the actual event can be a real anticlimax.

'I hadn't realized how warm they had kept the ward until I got home. The house seemed freezing and I wanted to suggest that we kept the central heating on all day, but I knew Liz was worried about the bills. And the children's noise... They were so pleased to have me back and of course expected me to play like I used to – and I just couldn't cope.'

'I thought my sleeping problems would be over when I got home, but in a way they were worse. If I was restless I was afraid that I would waken my husband with my tossing and turning, and he needed to be rested and alert for work the next day. I did suggest that I should sleep in the spare room for a while, but he wouldn't hear of it.'

'My friends from church were so excited that their prayers on my behalf had been answered that I felt honour-bound to be bright and cheerful every time they came to see me. I really didn't feel that well and yet I couldn't say so, because I felt as if I were letting them down. I know some of them were disappointed because I wasn't at church the first Sunday I was home.'

'It was strange, really. In hospital I got so tired of the people who could talk about nothing but their illness – and yet, when I got home, I really missed having someone to talk to who actually knew what it was like to have cancer. I was very glad when the secretary of the local cancer aftercare group called to see me. She had been in remission for four years and it really cheered me up.'

'When I had been out of hospital for two weeks, George caught bronchitis and he just went to bed and stayed there. It was awful. It was as if he was saying, "I've had enough – you're better now, so it's your turn to cope!" In the end my daughter had to leave her family and come and look after us both – I felt such a failure.'

It is easy to see from these remarks that the whole family will have adjustments to make. The patient often has unrealistic ideas about what they will be able to cope with, either expecting to do far more than is sensible or setting their sights unnecessarily low. The rest of the family may be banking on the fact that old roles will be taken up right away and that depression, pain and weakness will quickly be a thing of the past – and be disappointed if this does not happen. On the other hand, the patient may be longing to resume their previous responsibilities and their partner may be reluctant to allow them to do so – for all sorts of reasons. Either way, tension is likely to result. It is very natural to want to return to a familiar pattern of life immediately, but it is probably more realistic to regard the first two or three months at least as a transitional period and not to expect too much too soon – of anyone.

'Help! We're on our own!'
When Rebecca's mother was in hospital, the one thing Rebecca wanted above all else was to have her home again, so that she could look after her. But when the old lady was eventually discharged into her daughter's care, Rebecca panicked. There seemed to be so much to remember and so much to do, and her mother's lack of interest in food, far from being cured by home cooking, seemed to get worse.

'She wouldn't even try to use her arm on the mastectomy side, which meant that dressing and undressing was difficult and, as it was her right arm that was so stiff and sore, it made it hard for her to do much at all. Getting her to eat was a nightmare. She said that she would like one particular thing, and then an hour later, when I'd cooked it, she changed her mind and said that she just "couldn't fancy it". The dog got fatter, eating all her leftovers, and she got thinner. The worst times were when she said that she wished she was back in hospital and compared me unfavourably with the nurses. She seemed to have got so dependent on "the doctor says" or "nurse told me" for her confidence that if anyone who was not wearing a uniform or a white coat told her anything, she just ignored it.'

Fortunately for Rebecca (and for all of us), help was at hand in the form of the Community Healthcare Service. When someone is discharged from hospital, their own doctor is informed by letter. He or she will then either visit the patient at home or, if the patient is well enough, may ask them to visit the surgery. The doctor will also alert the district nurse (and the health visitor in the case of the under-fives or the elderly). If they are needed, the community physiotherapist, occupational therapist and social worker can also be called upon to assist the patient and their family.

The district nurse

The district nurse is a fully qualified and very experienced nurse whose job it is to look after anyone who needs nursing at home. If the patient comes out of hospital with stitches still in place, or dressings that need to be changed, she will come to the house to do this. She will be able to make suggestions about diet, and reluctant eaters will often be persuaded to eat when they know that the nurse has suggested a particular dish, even if they ignore the pleas of their nearest and dearest.

If the patient is well on the way to recovery, the district nurse will obviously not be needed to help for very long, but most of them like to build a relationship with the patient and their family so that, if care is needed at a later date, they are not strangers. This is particularly the case when a patient is in partial remission and may well need further treatment in the foreseeable future.

The district nurses I have met have almost all said the same things:

o Don't be afraid to ask for help. Even small worries can become enormous mountains if they are allowed to heap up on top of one another.

o We would prefer to get to know the patient when they are reasonably well, if this is possible. Then we are able to understand their needs better if their illness progresses.

o Don't feel that you have to handle any illness, and particularly cancer, in the way that you have seen Mrs X cope. No two people will have the same needs or the same inner resources.

o Time and resources are not unlimited and your district nurse cannot do everything. But she will know who else can help or give advice if you have any problems such as:

~the patient needs transport to get to the hospital for radiation treatment and cannot use public transport, but is not ill enough to need an ambulance

~there are financial problems which make it difficult for the patient to pay for fares to the hospital, or special dietary needs, appliances, prescriptions for medicines, etc.

~help with the housework is needed, or a midday meal because the patient is alone at home

~you just need someone to talk to or have any other worries.

Voluntary groups

In addition to the government funded assistance that we can call on, there are a number of voluntary or charitable groups, both national (see the list of useful addresses on page 188) and local. Cancer support groups at which those suffering with, or recovering from, cancer can meet and give mutual help and encouragement to each other are becoming increasingly common.

People vary in their need of such a group. Some are very glad to have another person to talk to who can identify with their feelings because they too have had cancer. Others just want to put the whole experience behind them, forget, if possible, that they have ever had the disease, and just get on with living. There is no right or wrong reaction – it is entirely a matter of personal choice. Relatives are often welcome at these groups too and, even if the patient does not want to be involved, it can often be very useful for first team supporters to get together and benefit from one another's experiences.

Sometimes we may want to ask questions and do not feel free to contact the doctor over what may seem a small point. This is where BACUP comes in. The British Association of Cancer United Patients (and their families and friends) is a cancer information service which was started by Dr Vicky Clement-Jones after she was treated for ovarian cancer (see page 125). The organization produces literature about the different forms of cancer, distributes its own newspaper and provides its own telephone counselling and question-answering service staffed by experienced cancer care nurses (see the list of useful addresses on page 188).

Follow-up appointments

After treatment for cancer, the patient will have regular check-ups with the hospital where they were treated. These will vary in frequency, depending on how satisfied the doctor is with progress. The first appointment after the patient is discharged will probably be arranged for a date some four to eight weeks after they have left hospital, and this first assessment can be a very stressful time for all those involved. The person most concerned is, of course, the one who has had the disease. They may be glad to be going to see the doctor because they are anxious to hear that they are 'doing well' and making good progress, but fearful that this may not be the case.

When my father came home from hospital his future outlook was not good, and he knew that. But denial was still influencing his thinking and he was somewhat frustrated by his lack of energy and slow progress towards the recovery he still hoped for. He pinned great hopes on his first follow-up appointment, feeling that the doctor would have some magic remedy for his weakness, or some new hope to offer. My mother had many anxieties about caring for him and questions that she was half afraid to ask. Put two people who are feeling like that in a busy outpatients clinic, surround them with old friends from the ward who are making rather better progress and are eager to compare notes, and you have the recipe for a very tense time.

Even if 'operation-mates' are doing less well than you or yours, there is a tendency to think 'will that be me (or him)... next time?' So those of us trying to keep the atmosphere positive and cheerful can be in a no-win situation.

Each time the news is good, the patient's confidence grows. But, even when the check-ups become part of a familiar routine, they are never completely stress-free. There is always the lurking question, 'Will it be all right *this* time?'

John felt as if he was playing Russian roulette every three months as he entered the hospital car park.

'I used to think to myself, "Is the bullet in the chamber this time?" and I would shake and sweat and feel physically sick. It was stupid really, because if I had got a recurrence it would not be made any worse or any bigger because the doctor discovered it was there. But I suppose I was operating on the "what you don't know can't hurt you" line of thinking.'

Pat Seed must have been one of the best-known cancer patients in Britain, since the appeal she started raised over £1,000,000 to buy a CAT scanner for cancer diagnosis at the Christie Hospital in Manchester. She readily confessed to hating her fortnightly visits. In *One Day at a Time* she wrote:

'Every couple of weeks Geoff and I drove from Garstang to the Christie. Each time we passed the high wire fencing before the Wythenshawe exit of the M63 motorway I felt as though cancer was closing in on me. I was no longer a person, but a patient... Coming back along the M63 knowing the medical report had been "so far, so good" gave a feeling of blessed relief. For another two weeks I could forget hospital.'

There is of course a positive side to hospital visits. If all is well, they become more widely spaced and this in itself is a confidence builder. It is also reassuring to know that an expert eye is being kept on the situation, so that the disease is unlikely to recur unnoticed. Check-up times are also an opportunity to ask questions, and although there tends to be a sense of time pressure if many other people are still waiting to be seen, we should not let that prevent us from raising any real problems. The doctor will himself probably ask whether the patient is:

o experiencing any pain

o having any difficulties with sleeping

o managing their appliance (if they have one) satisfactorily

o eating well and maintaining or gaining weight (a cancer sufferer is one of the few people who are glad to put on weight!)

o getting out and about and picking up the threads of a normal social life

o feeling ready to return to work or coping with the job done prior to becoming ill or, for someone based at home, able to look after home and family satisfactorily

o experiencing any sexual and/or emotional difficulties.

However, he may leave out the last three areas, either because he is in a hurry, or because the patient feels bound to give the impression that all is fine (whether it is or not), or simply because he forgets. We all know what it is like to have every intention of saying something quite important to a friend and then getting distracted by some unexpected turn in the conversation and forgetting all about it. If there are any problems that the doctor does not give us the opportunity to talk about, by asking a direct question, we should feel quite free to raise them – and this is where a written note to ourselves can often be a useful memory-jogger.

11 The loneliness of a long illness

'The biggest disease today is not leprosy or TB (or cancer), but rather the feeling of being unwanted, uncared for and deserted by everybody. The greatest evil is the lack of love... and the terrible indifference towards one's neighbour.'
MOTHER TERESA OF CALCUTTA

'Now that I was back amongst people I knew, I began to experience some of the peculiarities of society's response to cancer patients. Some people stick faithfully to the scapegoat ritual (one suffering for all the rest) and put as much distance between them and you as possible. Friends and acquaintances who would normally have rung up for a chat, popped in for a coffee, or called in on their way back from the shops, all of a sudden don't do any of those things. People who would erstwhile have greeted you with a hug and a kiss, now stand frozen to the spot a few feet away from you, blushing and stammering.

'There's another group of people who don't exclude you altogether, but include you in a way that marks you indelibly as the odd one out. These are the ones who, in a perfectly ordinary tone of voice, ask someone standing next to you how things are going, but feel obliged, when they turn to you, to narrow their eyes in conspiratorial pity, lower their voices to a whisper, and accompany the same question with a slow shake of the head.

'Cancer seems to evoke in the average man much the same emotions as it does in the people who have it: disgust, guilt, grief and of course that good old favourite, fear... I understand it now, but

I didn't understand it then. Just when I needed a lot of support and affection I had to cope with projected fear and rejection, which was hard.'

'I felt more alone once I was back at home than I had ever done in hospital. I couldn't think why this was until I realized that, now the immediate crisis was over, everyone else was simply getting on with their lives. I didn't blame them, I'd done it myself when friends had been bereaved. We had rallied round in the first few weeks, but then life's demands had taken over, fresh crises had occurred and the bereaved person was expected to cope and to "get over it" as best they could. The problem was that I wasn't at all sure that I *could* cope or that I *would* get over my cancer, and not one single person wanted to know that.'

'All through those grey blustery March days I was lashed by depression and overwhelming loneliness. It was as if the winds that were roaring through the trees and battering the daffodils into the mud were taking with them the last vestiges of the calmness and certainty about the future that I had managed to hang on to. Even the evidences of new life that were popping up everywhere in the garden, in spite of gales, seemed to mock rather than to encourage me. The worst part was that no one else could understand why I felt like that. After all, I was out of hospital and getting better, wasn't I? I couldn't explain and they couldn't understand and so I felt more isolated than ever.'

'I only went to the Good Friday service because its theme of suffering and death suited my mood. But it was there that something dawned on me that is so obvious to me now, and yet I had never grasped it before in years of church attendance. Jesus understands what this kind of agony is all about. In the garden of Gethsemane he was tortured by thoughts of what the future held: those he loved couldn't help him – they could not cope with any more emotional pressure themselves and blanked it out by going to sleep. And Jesus knew how I was feeling and he wanted to be with me in it; more than wanted to – could be – right where I was. As I reached out to take communion, I felt as if I was being wrapped around with total understanding and absolute love. The intensity of that experience has faded with time, but I have never again doubted that I am loved by God, and I know that I will never be abandoned.'

Any sense of being an outsider, an object of pity, a casualty who has been swept onto the sidelines by the onward rush of life, or simply someone who is 'not trying to be positive and get well', will inevitably make a person who is recovering from, or continuing to battle with, cancer feel very lonely. Of course, it is not done deliberately. People do not intend to be insensitive or unkind. But they are often bound by their own fears – fear of the disease, fear of doing or saying the wrong thing, and fear of getting involved in a situation they do not feel equipped to cope with.

Some close friends will probably quickly break through the barrier of 'what shall I say?' by visiting the patient in hospital. Others may have phoned or written before they get home and broken the ice that way. But for those who with considerable embarrassment confess, 'I haven't phoned/visited before because...

o I didn't want to bother you

o I didn't know what to say

o I just can't bear to think of... with cancer

o I thought they might be too poorly to chat on the phone

o I've had mother-in-law visiting/been working late at the office...'

we might suggest some of the following ideas, which will certainly make the patient (and their carers) feel less isolated.

Being there
Words of sympathy are not always the most meaningful thing – a hug or handshake speaks volumes. Be yourself and try to imagine what you would like to hear in the same situation. If you are of a gloomy disposition, think twice before you tell your friend too many horror stories about other people's illnesses. Be positive.

'The people who helped me most told me of others that they knew who had recovered from the same illness and now held down demanding jobs.'

Let the patient set the pace. If they want to talk about their illness – fine. If not, discuss the things you would have talked about before they were ill.

Phone calls can make a welcome break in a seemingly endless day, but beware of talking for too long, or keeping your friend standing up if the telephone is in the hall. It can be a good idea to suggest that the one who has been ill excuses themself when they are feeling tired, or tells you if they would prefer you to phone back at some other time. And do not be offended if they take you up on that offer.

Helping

Help is most often accepted if it is offered for specific things. Not 'Can I do anything for you?' but 'I am going into town to the bank and the supermarket – can I cash a cheque for you, or do some grocery shopping?'

If the patient is well enough, it is even better to invite them to come with you. But do remember that energy may well still be limited – and do not embark on a round of the sales!

Company and help offered together can be a real bonus.

'My kitchen drawers and cupboards were in a real muddle after so many "cooks" had been in the kitchen while I was in hospital. Margaret offered to help *me* to sort them out. She emptied the cupboards and put everything back. I cut shelf lining paper, decided what to throw away and told her where to put things. It was marvellous. I felt in control of my life for the first time for months, and when we had finished the kitchen seemed as if it was *mine* once more.'

Personal needs should not be overlooked either. After Eileen's mastectomy she was reluctant to shop for clothes, and found her friend's offer of a home shopping catalogue a great gift. All that Eileen had to do was make her choice – the owner of the catalogue did all the paperwork. Eileen tried the clothes on in the privacy of her own bedroom and was able to return anything that was unsuitable.

Helen did not want to buy new clothes, but she was painfully aware that her weight loss had made her skirts and dresses very badly fitting. Miss Evans was an elderly lady whose arthritic hip made it difficult for her to go shopping or do extra housework. But she was a very skilful seamstress. So her contribution to Helen's care was to offer to alter some of her clothes for her, 'leaving some of your favourites, dear, for when you have put those pounds back on again.' A very positive approach!

Hairdos for men and women can be done at home by those who have the required expertise (no pudding-basin jobs, please) and certainly boost morale. Being included in the normal life of the community, even if you can only do a fraction of what you did before, has the same effect. But friends should beware of appearing to make takeover bids.

When Colin came out of hospital, he was aware that he needed to rebuild his relationship with his eight- and ten-year-old sons, and he got very frustrated because well-meaning friends kept inviting them out, to 'give you some peace and quiet'. Families need time apart, but they also need time to be together – on their own.

Supporting

People need praying *for* just as much when they are at home as when they are in hospital. And, because concentration is often poor when you are feeling weak and tired, an offer to read and pray *with* someone is often very much appreciated. If someone at the church records the Sunday services, a tape can make you feel part of what is going on once again. And even if a convalescent person feels a bit daunted by listening to a whole service, they can be encouraged to listen a bit at a time.

Here again, being asked to help others can be a great relief to someone who has been on the receiving end of care for weeks or months.

Judy had been a member of a 'prayer chain' before she was ill. This meant that in an emergency she would be phoned and asked to pray for the needy person or situation and then to ring the next person in the chain and ask them to do the same. Judy knew that the other members of the chain had prayed for her many times when she was in hospital. The day the phone rang and she was asked to pray for a friend's sick grandchild was a turning point in her own recovery.

'Maria didn't even ask how I was. Suddenly I was just like everyone else, ordinary, coping, and expected to have something to contribute. It was fantastic. I felt as if my life started to get back to normal from that point on and, although there have been a few hiccoughs along the way, I've never really looked back.'

What about the workers?
It is not just the patients who can feel lonely in their illness – the first team supporters may well feel very isolated too. There are all sorts of reasons for this. When someone is diagnosed as having cancer, everyone tries to be loving and supportive, and that is as it should be. But the relatives and close friends are deeply involved in the cancer crisis too, and almost as deeply in need of support. Unfortunately those a little further removed from the situation often fail to recognize this, especially if we manage to give the impression that we are coping quite well, thank you.

Catherine is a midwife who gives the impression of having everything totally under control. When her husband developed cancer, she seemed to absorb the problem and carry on with her faith and serenity unruffled. Her friends were loud in their praise for the wonderful way she coped, but within the privacy of their home she and her husband were finding things very far from easy.

'Gerry's personality seemed to change as a result of his chemotherapy. He always had a hasty temper, but after his treatment he seemed to have no self-control at all. He said that he would give the treatment three months and, if he was not better by then, he would commit suicide. It was all or nothing as far as he was concerned. Outwardly nothing had changed – he was still the genial churchwarden and I was the village midwife who brought babies into the world and whose days were full of life, not death... but I felt as if I was walking along a precipice. One false step could spell disaster. The strain was terrible because Gerry would not tell *anyone* how he felt. We were both putting up an act in public, but in private... Then one day (after a particularly difficult week) a friend asked me if I felt all right, because I looked pale – and instead of brushing it aside as I would normally have done, I burst into tears all over her. I didn't think I'd ever stop crying. Fortunately she wasn't put off by my sudden character change, but took me home and plied me with tea and sympathy. It was fantastic to have someone hold *me* in her arms for a change instead of me trying to prop up my entire world.'

You could say that it was Catherine's own fault that she was under such strain, but if people cast you in a certain role, it is very hard to step out of it. And few of us find it easy to ask for help, or to admit that a close relationship which is under threat anyway is in danger of disintegrating. Hard though it may be to let others know what is happening, desperate times call for desperate measures. We need to sink our pride for the sake of everyone concerned.

If we are living with the cancer sufferer, we can also feel cut off from normal life simply because he or she *is* ill. People who are recovering from surgery, radiation or chemotherapy often feel tired and depressed, and simply do not want to talk or to entertain visitors. It is hard to feel free to go out and do anything but the bare minimum of things that have to be done – to enjoy ourselves can seem almost like a betrayal. And yet this situation can go on for months at a time. Faced with this problem, what should we do?

o We should stop feeling guilty because we are healthy and our loved one has cancer.

o We should realize that we are probably their main link with the outside world, and if we have something new and interesting to talk about because we have done something we enjoy, or been involved with an area of life outside the 'cancer situation', we are bringing something of positive value into the home. (We need to balance this, of course, against the problem of making them feel that we are simply getting on with our life without them.)

o We should accept that we cannot give out indefinitely unless we also take in. So, apart from allowing ourselves to take opportunities we may be given to go out and do things that we enjoy, we need to eat properly, sleep adequately, and take some time each day to relax physically and to take in emotionally and spiritually.

These may sound ludicrous suggestions if you are in the heavy nursing stage, and certainly it will be very much more difficult (although just as essential) then, but in any except the most pressured times it is a matter of priorities. We can choose how to spend that spare twenty minutes which we may have in the middle of the day.

Will we lie down on the settee, or clean underneath it?

Will we walk to the shops and enjoy the sunshine, or rush along in the car?

Will we prepare a snack and set a tray for ourselves with as much care as we would for the invalid, or nibble a biscuit as we rush through yet another chore?

We may have a problem persuading ourselves that we are justified in doing this for ourselves. If all else fails, we can tell ourselves that it is ultimately for the patient's benefit, which it certainly will be.

Love never fails

Loneliness is not the only emotional pitfall which those of us who are 'living with cancer' may tumble into – there can be an awful lot of anger bubbling away under the surface as well. Not all of it is as dramatic as Catherine's husband and his threat of suicide; it can demonstrate itself in petty little ways. Often patients will cheerfully agree to do anything that the medical team suggests, but pour scorn on a similar idea that originates from those closest to them. This can be very annoying as well as very upsetting, making the would-be helpers feel rejected and unloved, and leading to some very bitter arguments.

Rebecca felt that her mother was being totally unreasonable, and blaming her for everything that went wrong in the day – they argued as they had not done since Rebecca was a teenager. Eventually Rebecca confided in the health visitor and was very relieved to hear that hers was by no means an unusual situation.

'Your mother doesn't behave like this with other people,' she reassured Rebecca, 'because she does not feel secure enough with them to take the risk. It may seem twisted and all wrong, but your mother is actually showing how very safe she feels with you, by allowing her anger to surface. Hang on to that fact, if you can, and also realize that you are both having to adjust to new roles – you are the parent figure now and your mother is the dependent one, which is hard for both of you to accept. It will be much easier to be more tolerant and to take the flare-ups in your stride if you relax, knowing that the basic love between you is not really threatened.'

It can sound very simple, put like that, by someone who is emotionally detached from the situation, but there will be times for all of us when we wonder how much further we can go before we reach the end of our tether.

Elizabeth and Madeleine were friends who shared a flat very happily together for a long time before Madeleine developed cancer. They weathered the storms of the early treatment together and enjoyed the periods of remission that Madeleine had. Eventually, though, the disease began to progress, and both women had to struggle with their questions about what the future might hold and their ability to cope with it. Tension grew and their relationship became a battleground.

'Hanging on the bathroom door (of all places) was a poster bearing a beautiful paraphrase of 1 Corinthians 13, that great Christian hymn about love. One day, after a particularly tempestuous row, I found it lying on my bedroom floor where Mads had flung it in a rage... an eloquent message that hit me hard... On another occasion when Madeleine seemed very unreasonable, I was so furious I stormed out of the flat and walked round trying to cool off... I felt so angry that when I came back I hurled a small suitcase across my room, hoping that Mads would realize how impossible I was finding the situation.

'The questions that pounded through my mind were to do with practicalities. I knew I had no direct responsibility for Madeleine... illness, death and bereavement came to relatives – and of course you had no choice but to go through with it. But I had a choice. I didn't want to leave... the bond which had been established between us over the previous ten years made it unthinkable to walk out. How could I say, even if I wanted to, "Since it is clear that you are dying, I hope you will understand that I must move out; after all, I have my own life to live"? Yet could I cope with what lay ahead?... supposing I cracked, what then?

'I was visiting my parents... for a long weekend and had the opportunity to slip off and walk along the cliffs at Hope Cove – a name which in retrospect seems symbolic. In my anxiety and

confusion I asked God to show me clearly what he wanted me to do...
I needed some very definite word of guidance. With amazing force
the words of the poster which had been flung onto my bedroom floor
came into my mind:

"Love bears all things, believes all things, hopes all things,
endures all things. Love never ends."

'I walked back along those cliffs with a curious sense of elation,
and an awareness that the burden of uncertainty had been lifted from
me. The situation was unchanged, but my perspective was changed,
and I knew without a doubt where I was going: my resources were
inadequate and my human capacity to love limited, but Christ's love
working in and through me would be sufficient. Whatever lay ahead,
I would be given the divine resources which would get us both
through.

'Does this sound unrealistic or trite? I can only say that in the four
months that remained for Madeleine, and long after her death, the
sense of God's love working in the situation was often almost
overwhelming.'

Was Elizabeth given special treatment? An extraordinary degree of
help for an unusually difficult situation? I do not think so. Many
other people have experienced exactly the same sense of the care and
compassion of God, although the detailed way in which that support
has been given has obviously been different.

When I was at school, one of our end-of-term treats was to play
'Shipwreck' in the gym. This was a wild and wonderful game which
involved getting out all the pieces of apparatus and swinging between
them on the ropes. If you fell off, you were drowned or eaten by
sharks. It was very hard to stay on the ropes after a while, because
your arms became extremely tired. But the streetwise members of the
class knew what to do – they tied a knot at the end of the rope and put
their feet on it.

This, in a sense, is what Elizabeth did. She simply recognized her
limitations and when she came to the end of her rope she tied a knot
and hung on. The critical part of the whole operation was that she
tied her knot by depending completely on God's love and not her own
– or anyone else's – resources. And she proved, as have many others
who have put it to the test, that God's love never fails.

12 Facing the long march

There certainly is a large element of picking yourself up, dusting yourself down and starting all over again when it comes to living with cancer. With the sophistication of today's treatment methods, and because new ways of dealing with the disease are constantly being discovered, many patients, even if they are not officially pronounced 'cured', can have treatment, enjoy a period of complete or partial remission, have another session of treatment, recover and carry on again in the same way for long periods of time. When this happens, it is very much a case of learning to live with a disease – guerrilla warfare perhaps, rather than one all-out conclusive battle.

Guerrilla fighters are slippery customers. One of their most powerful weapons is the element of surprise and the fear that this generates. If you live in a country where there is political unrest and guerrilla warfare, you can never relax. When you travel, you have always to be on your guard. You never know who your enemy is or where he will strike next.

The plus factor
Living with cancer can be much the same. The fear of recurrence can shadow our lives, if we allow it to do so, but there *is* another way to handle it. In one of the Chinese dialects the symbol for the word 'crisis' is made up of two other symbols: 'danger' and 'opportunity'. There is certainly danger inherent in having cancer, but there is also a tremendous opportunity for personal growth and character development. So much so that many patients (and their families) actually reach a point where they say that they are glad they have had

to deal with the disease because of the changes it has brought into their lives.

Jo Hilton was one of those people. She wrote:

'Do I sound like Pollyanna when I say that I am *glad* that I have cancer? Of course I cannot be glad of the pain that it has brought to my nearest and dearest, but in spite of all that, I am really and truly happy that it happened this way. It has brought me so many friends... I never knew before how much I was loved... I did not know how kind my neighbours could be. I did not know the meaning of the words cherish, comfort and cancer. They were only words, but now I have experienced them all.

'The hymn "God moves in a mysterious way" was one of my grandmother's favourites. She quoted lines from it with such confidence that even I, the most timid and fearful of all her many grandchildren, received courage from the well-worn words. When I cowered in terror because of a thunderstorm she used to make me repeat the verse:

Ye fearful saints, fresh courage take,
The clouds ye so much dread
Are big with mercy, and shall break
In blessings on your head.

'It has taken cancer to make me realize to the full the truth of those words. As a small child I was always afraid... afraid I would be ill, miss the promised treat, the party, the concert. Sure enough I always was, but pain and sickness when they came did not worry me at all... it was the *fear* of them that cast black shadows over my childhood.

'In adult life cancer was my secret hidden fear... the unmentionable thing only spoken of in whispers. And yet from the moment the specialist spoke the dreaded word and I knew that it applied to me I have been released from all fears, both great and small. I am not afraid of anything... of life – of death... and these three years have been the happiest of my life. I have so many blessings it is impossible to count them, and it seems incredible that I should have spent so long in fear and ignorance.'

Jo described her life as 'living with cancer' rather than dying from it.

'In twenty-three years I have had six years altogether when we hoped I was cured, but never for a sufficiently long period for the doctors to say I was cured, and so I have learned to live one day at a time.'

For Jo it was release from fear and the fact that she has experienced the love and compassion of others which have made her experience of cancer so valuable, and that is by no means uncommon. A patient who was being cared for very lovingly in a hospice said to one of the nurses, 'All my life I have been nobody, worth nothing to anyone, but here I am someone special.'

Another common bonus, in the opinion of many patients, is a new appreciation of family and friends and a realization of the importance of letting them know that they are appreciated. There is a sense of not wanting to postpone pleasure and enjoying their company *today*. It is true that some relationships founder under the pressure of an illness like cancer, but many others go from strength to strength, and some that were beginning to run into rough weather have been steadied and put back on course.

Penny Brohn felt very strongly that her cancer had been triggered off by a long period of emotional psychological stress. She also believed that if her body was to get well again, the underlying problems had to be dealt with.

'My certainty, now absolute, that my tumour would never be overcome except by a total cleansing of myself presented me with a dilemma. Like most married couples, David and I had accumulated our fair share of junk over the years which we had carefully been brushing under the carpet and assiduously trying to ignore... I had no doubt that a long overdue spring clean was an essential prerequisite to the course of treatment on which I was about to embark; the dilemma existed only because I was afraid... If things went wrong I could see myself adding so much more to the burden I was already carrying – a marriage on the rocks, for example.

'As it turned out, I need not have feared. David proved to be just as keen as I was to undertake this exposure, and we lay together in the darkness... and played a grown-up version of the children's game 'Truth, Dare, Kiss or Promise' until way into the night.

'Instead of the hours of accusations and recriminations that I had anticipated with such dread, we found ourselves capable of real forgiveness and understanding... We were able to jump off the treadmill of "But you always..." and "That's because you never..." For once we managed not to justify our own weaknesses and failures on the basis of being married to someone who was even worse. We started to accept and forgive each other.

'I am one of the many people who say they are glad they had cancer... The indescribable sweetness and joy of that night and the peace that came from it was so beautiful a consequence of being hit by a virtually incurable disease that I can honestly say it was worth it!

'Naturally we thought that we had solved all our problems with one fantastic stroke and imagined... that we would proceed in total harmony and understanding, with lots of laughingly tolerant generosity of spirit swilling round us for the rest of our days. Of course we had done no such thing, but we had hacked a way through the jungle of thorns that had grown up around us, and the Sleeping Beauty of our precious marriage was at least awake again.'

The experience of having cancer tests people in many ways, and that is certainly true in the area of faith. We often have to experience the 'dark night of the soul' as Christians from earlier centuries called it – doubt, depression and sometimes even despair – before we come to a place where hope, trust and love seem possible again. But those who do so are adamant that it has been an experience they value greatly.

'My faith has been like an anchor holding me steady in spite of the storm. I always used to be afraid that I would falter and let God down if the going got difficult, and sometimes that has seemed to be a distinct possibility. But the anchor has held me (I haven't held it) and now I know that if I can be kept through this experience, I can be kept through anything.'

'I had to reassess everything – my attitude to other people, myself and to God. I had to ask myself what I was basing my life on – truth or wishful thinking? I went through agonies, but now "I *know* whom I have believed and am convinced that he is able to guard what I have entrusted to him," and that certainly is a treasure beyond price.'

'I learned to really trust God, in spite of not being able to understand, in a way that one doesn't when everything is running smoothly.'

'I know that my cancer has cemented my relationship with God. I have now experienced God the Father as provider, God the Spirit as comforter, and God the Son, Jesus, not only as saviour, but also as the ultimate and supreme friend. What a friend I have in him.'

'Teach us to number our days aright that we may gain a heart of wisdom.' Cancer has a habit of making us 'number our days', but one of the major secondary gains of having the disease – or facing it within the family – is the discovery many people make about living one day at a time.

The idea of living in the present is typified by Pat Seed. She was diagnosed as having an ovarian tumour. The problem was quite widespread and the doctors faced her bluntly with the fact that she probably had only months to live (in fact she survived for a number of years). Undaunted, she made up her mind that she would live every day to its fullest, come what may.

'Does it come as a surprise to know that in spite of having been told that I am dying, I am happy? That's no heroic statement. It's true... Death itself doesn't frighten me. I regard it merely as the shedding of the form I will no longer require in the life to follow. And if I am wrong, and there isn't a life after our life here on earth, then it won't matter anyway...

'If I am afraid I am not going to live my life to the full, I am not going to enjoy the good things for fear they may end or be taken away from me... So I have cancer. I am surrounded by a kind and loving family... yet they cannot have cancer for me. That is something I have to do by myself. And sitting wondering whether today, tomorrow or the day after tomorrow might be my last isn't going to change a thing. It will only prevent me from making the most of today...'

Whether you've been told that you are dying of cancer or that you can expect to live for another sixty years, no human being can live for more than one day at a time. Whatever circumstances we are faced with, *this* day is the only day in which we can deal with them effectively. The New Testament puts it as a simple truth: 'Why worry about tomorrow, when today has sufficient cares of its own?' Like many other simple truths, its very simplicity causes it to be overlooked, underestimated, ignored... Yet it is a basic ingredient of happiness.

Some time ago I came across the following lines. I wish I had thought of these wise words, but I can learn from them.

This is the beginning of a new day.
God has given me this day to use as I will.
I can waste it or use it for good.
What I do today is important, for I am
Exchanging a day of my life for it.
When tomorrow comes this day will be gone for ever,
Leaving in its place something that I have traded for it.
I want it to be gain, not loss;
Good, not evil;
Success, not failure, in order that I shall not regret
The price I paid for it.

Unfinished business

'I have finished the work you gave me to do' (Jesus' words recorded in John's gospel). One of the most difficult aspects of a premature death to come to terms with is the sense of having unfinished business left behind you.

'I often used to wonder why I had been so frantic with fear and anxiety when I first knew how ill I was. After all, with my spiritual beliefs I wasn't afraid of being dead, and although I didn't fancy the actual process of dying, it hardly seemed to justify all the emotion that had been aroused in me...

'I began to see that the real truth about my fear of dying had a lot to do with David and the children. In common with many other people I had a personal model of what "wonderful wives" and "marvellous mothers" were like, but I was still in the rehearsal stage, I hadn't quite made mine a star performance yet, so I simply wasn't ready to die. I didn't yet have enough stability or security in my roles as wife and mother to be ready to relinquish them. There was too much left to be done, too much that was unfinished.'

It is not just in the area of marriage and parenthood that people feel that they have unfinished business to complete – although this is very common. Personal goals, business commitments and wider relationships can all present the same challenge. And the fact that a prolonged battle with cancer is necessary often provides the impetus for us to grapple with these issues, rather than leaving them until it is too late.

'The cancer, with its implicit threat of death, was forcing us to deal with the unfinished business that usually gets clumped together at the end of the marriage agenda, turning up, like as not, when there's no time left to deal with it. Knowing that we couldn't assume anything about the time available to us, we were trying to get on with this now... I wanted to feel free to die without guilt about my shortcomings as a wife, and David had to feel able to let me die without blaming himself for his performance as a husband. We were trying to get it right *now*, not in some mythical future that might never come.'

The process of completing unfinished business is never easy. In fact it may be very painful to say 'I'm sorry,' or to expose your inner feelings so that a relationship can be healed. Some people find they rethink their lives completely and decide to live very differently – not just because they do not know how much longer they might have to accomplish what is important to them, but because what is important to them changes in the light of a possibly limited lifespan.

'I have decided that life is for living and the mundane chores can wait.'

'I have become less worried about what people think of me or what I achieve in terms of success as I used to measure it. I have suddenly discovered the freedom to be myself, the desire to give something of value to my generation and the determination to invest my life – whether it is long or short – in something that will live for ever... and for me that *has* to be spiritual values. I am utterly convinced that

I shall be given enough time and enough strength to do that. Jesus only had an active ministry of three years. He died a young man at thirty-three. But before he died his last words were, "It is finished," and that is what I want to be able to say.'

Painful, challenging and taxing it may be, but to all of us who have grasped the opportunity of dealing with unfinished business comes an unshakable sense of completion and contentment, whatever difficulties may still remain. And the freedom that comes from the very fact of having grappled with something that was painful and threatening, even if it is not totally resolved, often allows the patient to concentrate on their physical needs with an unfettered mind. Elisabeth Kübler-Ross explains it like this.

'When a patient has no unfinished business there is a sense of peace and harmony, a sense of having done what needed to be done. It is like a housewife who has put her children to bed at night. The dishes are washed... the dining room table is cleared and she has a sense of having done everything she wanted to do and has planned to do that day... She has a sense of pride, a feeling of accomplishment and it is okay now for her to go to sleep. That, in the simplest words I know, is the finishing of unfinished business.'

Goals

Discovering how much you are loved. Being released from the fear of the future. Finding that your faith *will* hold in a time of trial. Living every day to its limits. Seeing relationships restored. Gaining a new perspective on what is important in life. These are all positive parts of the long march with cancer that many of us have experienced in whole or in part. But of course they do not all happen instantly. In the early days it is often a fight for emotional survival from one milestone to the next.

'My doctor told me to go home and start setting small goals for the future. Even something as simple as beginning to read some of the lengthy books that I had "always meant to get down to", believing that I would live long enough to finish them, was a step in the right direction.'

Goals are important for living life to the full at every stage, and this is particularly so in the face of life-threatening disease. Goals not only give a shape and purpose to life, but when they are accomplished they give an enormous morale boost and sense of being in control of one's circumstances at a time when so much is out of control.

For many patients, at the beginning of their recovery period, getting home from hospital or surviving the radiation treatment or chemotherapy are major goals. But once they are safely behind them, more tangible milestones are often important. They may be relatively small or simple things:

o Beth was determined that she was going to live long enough to write a magazine article about her experiences.

o George wanted to complete the dolls' house that he had started to make for his granddaughter before he became ill.

o Mary decided that she would fight her way through the winter so that she would see the swallows return to their nests under her eaves.

Sometimes they are more ambitious:

o Ophelia decided that since one of the first things God did on this earth was to create a garden, she would make it her goal to make one as a gift to those who would live in her home after her. (Just in case she did not see her plants come to maturity she wrote it all down in a book, so that her successors in the house would not dig things up before they had had the chance to discover what was there.)

o Joy was utterly convinced that she would stay well for long enough to visit her daughter in Australia – and she did.

And some goals have a life-changing impact on thousands of other people, just because one person decided to use their remaining days, months or years to change the world a little – even when it seemed totally over-ambitious even to try.

Dr Vicky Clement-Jones went into hospital to have an abscess drained and awoke from the anaesthetic to discover that instead of an abscess the surgeon had discovered advanced ovarian cancer. The situation was so serious that she was told she probably had only months to live. Not surprisingly, she was devastated and angry. In the days that followed she realized that being a doctor offered no protection against the emotional trauma of cancer, and she had little idea of how to cope with the disease from the patient's side of the blankets.

'Well, Vicky,' she thought to herself, 'if you're going to die in three months, you're going to get something positive out of this.' She did not die and, in spite of fourteen months of major surgery and debilitating chemotherapy treatment, she did make something very positive out of her experience. Realizing how little information was available for patients and their families she set up the information and counselling service BACUP. This feat of organization and liaison with various medical bodies and charities took a year, and for much of that time Vicky herself was having further treatment as a recurrence of the disease was discovered. But her determination to make sure that her experience was not wasted kept her going, and her vision became a reality in October 1985.

In its first year BACUP brought comfort, counsel and accurate information to more than 13,000 cancer patients, their families and friends – all because one woman set a goal for what looked like the last few weeks of her life. Perhaps because of her determination to make something positive out of her illness, Vicky Clement-Jones had stretched those three months to four years when she died in 1987. But she did so knowing that thousands of people had already benefited because she had come face to face with cancer.

Pat Seed, whom we have also mentioned earlier, was another victim of ovarian cancer who was given a very gloomy prognosis. With the hope of gaining more than the six months of life that the doctors forecast for her, she embarked on radiotherapy treatment, and it was during her stay in hospital for that treatment that her goal was set. One night she could not sleep and she went in search of the ward kitchen and a cup of tea. She got lost and ended up in the kitchen of the children's ward.

'Tiptoeing past the cots and the little beds I was filled with a cold fury that little children such as these should be stricken with cancer. Any self-pity I might have been feeling went out of the window and along with the anger was a sense of helplessness. Oh, if only one could do something – but what?'

During Pat's visits to the outpatients department of the Christie Hospital she had heard about the CAT scanner and its enormous usefulness in helping doctors to diagnose certain types of tumour and pinpoint them for accurate treatment. At that time, though, the Christie, even though it was a specialist cancer hospital, did not possess a scanner of its own. A few patients each week were able to make use of Manchester University Medical School's scanner, but the doctors reckoned that at least half of the 5,000 cancer patients they dealt with each year could benefit from the CAT's diagnostic abilities. The problem was that these machines are extremely expensive, the National Health Service could not provide the (then) £500,000 needed to buy one, and the 1948 Health Act prevented appeals for money being made direct to the general public by the hospital.

Pat Seed made her goal a CAT scanner for the Christie Hospital. She was a wife, a mother and a journalist – in that order! If she had only six months to live, she wanted to spend as much time as she could with her family and, having worked for a while as the secretary to the North-West Regional Director of the Missions to Seamen, she knew just how time-consuming it was to run a charitable body. In any case, she reasoned, how could one woman, who was in poor health anyway, hope to raise £500,000?

She wrestled with the problem for some time and then came to a decision. She was facing an enemy now every bit as lethal as a soldier with a gun in his hand. She had survived the Second World War – now she would survive her attack of cancer at least for long enough to get an appeal launched. And with that she set out determinedly on her 'Scanner Trail'.

Speaking five years later, Pat said that if she had known at the beginning what lay ahead, she would have died there and then – out of fright, not from cancer! As it was, although the cost trebled so that the final target became £1.5 million, Pat worked on undaunted, travelling, writing, speaking and driving herself through a sixteen-hour working day, living one day at a time and inspiring thousands of other people to join her. Less than three years later, the vision became a reality. The Christie's own scanner, housed in its own building, began to work for the benefit of cancer patients in northwest England.

Penny Brohn opted for an unconventional way of dealing with her breast cancer. Convinced that the tumour was the outward symptom of inward turmoil, she rejected the proposed mastectomy in favour of an approach that would treat her as a whole person rather than simply a diseased breast. Unable to find support or encouragement from doctors in England, she went to Dr Josef Issels' clinic in Bavaria. As she battled through the treatment, far away from family and friends and struggling with a foreign language, loneliness and fear as well as the disease itself, she too set her goal.

She made up her mind that if there were others who wanted to handle their cancer in the way that she had wanted to cope with hers, she would help them. Back home in England she would work with others to set up a centre for the holistic treatment of cancer – taking the mind, emotions and spirit into account, as well as the body.

It was another enormous undertaking. But from small beginnings in someone's home, one day a week, Penny's vision became a reality. The Bristol Cancer Help Centre's own building was opened in 1983 by Prince Charles, and Penny worked there for many years, sharing her love and her insights with other patients.

More recently art dealer Sara Davonport bought a dilapidated Welsh Presbyterian church, just off Fulham Broadway in west London, and founded the Haven. She had been shocked when her children's nanny had been sent home after a diagnosis of breast cancer, with little support, counselling or discussion about the disease. The idea was to create a space as unlike a hospital as possible, where women could support one another and find information advice and services not available elsewhere.

Eleanor Meade is someone else who is determined that something good should come out of her experience of breast cancer. When she was advised to have a mastectomy she opted for reconstruction of her breast as part of the same procedure – an operation that took nine hours, and initially left her arm on the affected side with very limited movement. After her operation she had three very brief visits from a physiotherapist, who gave her a sheet of exercises and left her to get her arm moving again as best she could. Eleanor devised her own scheme of exercises, using a basic fitness video by Rosemary Conley. This worked well up to a point, but when, several months later, her surgeon told her that as long as she could do up her bra and comb her hair she should consider that 'good enough', Eleanor was incensed. She was determined not to accept anything less than full function. She wanted to be like any other forty-three-year-old woman, and when she discovered that many other women had had even less help than she had in regaining movement and preventing swelling in their arms after their surgery, she decided that something had to be done.

'It may sound weird, but I felt that I had built up a relationship with Rosemary while I did her exercises,' said Eleanor. 'I used to talk back to the video and felt that I had a warm and encouraging friend in the room with me.' It was this sense of support that gave her the inspiration for the next step. If ordinary exercises had helped her so much, surely a video of exercises specially designed to be used after breast surgery would be a great asset to other women going through the trauma of the diagnosis of, and recovery from, breast cancer?

A short while later Eleanor met Rosemary Conley at a health farm, where the diet and fitness expert was running a series of classes, and, greatly daring, asked if she would consider appearing on such a video. At first Rosemary was dubious about the financial viability of such an undertaking, but Eleanor is very persuasive. When she explained that her husband ran a video company and so could cover the expense involved in actually producing it, Rosemary agreed to donate her time and teach the exercises. She also offered the services of her choreographer, who would devise a programme of graduated movement under the guidance of a specialist breast cancer physiotherapist.

As the project developed, Eleanor realized that it might also be helpful for ordinary women to share their experience of facing up to and dealing with the disease, and so the exercise video became a double album, entitled 'Fight Back and Get Fit'. One tape features a group of women and their partners, discussing the impact of breast cancer in their lives, and the other has exercises with which the patient can become familiar before her operation, which can be begun immediately after surgery and take the women right through their recovery period.

These examples all happen to come from Britain. But there are many in other parts of the world who have approached their cancer in equally determined fashion.

Big goals, small goals – it's not the size that is important, but the impetus they give to our lives. For we need constantly to bear in mind that, after treatment for cancer, most people still have a lot of living to do. And those of us who are caring for them need to have our goals for that care clearly in our minds.

Of course, how much the patient will be able, or want, to do will depend on how completely the cancer has been dealt with. We cannot make that decision for them. But, far from pushing the cancer sufferer too far, most of us tend to protect and protest too much. Our goal for ourselves and the patient should be to care for him or her in such a way that we regain the greatest degree of normality possible and live the life that remains – whether it be long or short – as fully as we can.

This means that we will not:

o be overprotective

o cope with life so well that the patient feels redundant

o be negative about any progress, no matter how slow it may seem to us

o discourage the patient from setting demanding goals

o tell patients that they cannot do things, but let them discover their limits for themselves

o deter patients from assuming responsibility for themselves, their work and their lifestyle as soon as they are able

o cling on to any of the patient's roles that we may have had to assume, if they want to take them on again.

Attitude is vitally important at this, as in any other, stage of the cancer war. The point is graphically illustrated by the true story of two men who were both discharged from hospital with a life expectancy of six months.

The first went home, organized his affairs, said goodbye to his relations, retired to bed and died two weeks later.

The other man looked at his brood of noisy, quarrelsome children and at his harassed wife and braced himself. 'She'll never cope with this lot on her own,' he said to himself, 'and I'm blowed if I want her marrying again. I'd better make sure I'm around till they grow up.' And twenty years later, he is!

13 Where is God when it hurts?

'It is not as a child that I believe and confess Jesus Christ. My "hosanna" is born of a furnace of doubt.'
FYODOR DOSTOEVSKY

One of the things that I found hardest to handle about my father's illness was the spiritual turmoil that it tossed me into – so I make no excuse for concentrating in this section on problems which loom particularly large for those who share my Christian faith. Always a questioner by nature, the stream of whys and what ifs swirled around me like an angry torrent. I felt as if I were marooned on a rock in the middle of a river, and the only way to get back to the safety of the shore was to build a bridge of answers. The problem was that no sooner did I get one plank hammered firmly into place than it seemed to get swept away again by the next rush of water.

One of the biggest hindrances to getting the bridge started at all was the attitude of so many of my friends, who simply did not seem to see that there could be a problem – or if they did, they refused to admit it.

'You are a committed Christian. Your parents are committed Christians. Christians know that there is nothing to fear about death, so I'm sure that you will all cope wonderfully.'

These were the actual words spoken to me by someone who should have known better. Looking back, I can see now that he was probably protecting himself from an emotional involvement that he felt unable to handle. If we had not coped, he might have had to, and perhaps...? Whatever his reasons for trying to push us into this mould, it made me feel more confused than I was already. Should Christians not grieve, then? Should they just accept a supposedly terminal illness as 'God's will' and/or a test of faith? What *could* we expect from God? What *should* we ask him for?

The situation was further complicated – to my mind – by my father's attitude. A couple of years before he was ill, he had said to me:

'I don't want anyone crying for me when I am gone. I know where I am going and I know that what awaits me there is even better than what I've got now. And that,' he concluded with his usual cheery grin, 'is pretty good.'

Of course I protested that we would certainly cry because we loved him and would miss him, but, as is often the way of such conversations, we quickly passed on to happier and seemingly more important topics, and the subject was not mentioned again until a few weeks before his cancer was diagnosed. Grappling with his own sadness when his younger brother died very suddenly from post-operative complications following his surgery for stomach cancer, my father said:

'When God crooks his finger and says, "Come in, number nine, your time is up," and you're in that boat, there isn't a thing that you or I can do about it.'

And this, ultimately, was his attitude towards his own illness. Very little obvious denial, a more marked degree of depression and withdrawal, and an apparent quiet acceptance that this was to be the way of things. It should have been a comfort, but actually it faced me with a lot more questions. If he was accepting it, then who was I to do otherwise? Could I, should I, fight for life on his behalf? After all, he still had so much to give to others, so much to do for God, and he was so much loved that his death was unthinkable, even if he had already enjoyed seventy-two action-filled years. But the question lingered on... was it unthinkable to God and out of his purposes?... or was it *my* potential loss that I was refusing to face?

And even if I could accept cancer as a way of death for someone who was older, where was God when a college friend lost her leg through cancer, a two-year-old developed a kidney tumour, and a man of God like David Watson, who had helped thousands to find faith, was taken out of action by malignant disease in his bowel and liver? Why heal others when *these* lives, which held so much potential, were not restored? I just did not understand it, and as my perplexity grew, it seemed as if my little rock of faith was in danger of getting totally submerged.

Never being one to admit defeat easily, I let God know that I had some questions and I needed answers – now! Of course, it did not happen quite like that, but as I prayed, read, poured my heart out to people who had faced the same situation, and battered those who had a greater understanding of the Christian faith than I have with my questions and doubts, a bridge was built. I cannot say that it was a totally solid construction. The planks of certainty had – and still have – large gaps of 'don't know' between them, and without the ropes of faith which eventually lashed them together it would have been a very fragile structure – but it held.

We all have a different sized gap to span over this particular river. For some it is the merest ditch; for others it is more of a mini-ocean. But I have met very few people who have actually been through the cancer crisis who have not had some problems to face in this area. So, for those who are currently in the business of bridge construction, let me share some of the building materials which I found would do the job, in the hope that they will at least give something to work with.

o It is not wrong to ask questions.

If God had wanted zombies to inhabit the earth he would have made us differently. He gave us our minds and enabled us to think, question and discover. Jesus gasped out the biggest question of all as he hung on the cross, 'My God, my God, why have you forsaken me?' God had spoken audibly before, during the three years of Jesus' ministry, but we have no record of an answer to this desperate cry. And perhaps this says something to us in our search for reasons. We may ask the question, but we have no right to demand an answer. Sometimes one will be given, if it is necessary for us to know. At other times we may simply have to accept that there is an answer, although God has not given it – and since all God's dealings with us are loving and for our ultimate good, we can leave the matter there. This is where faith comes in.

o God did not promise a rose garden.

Some people have a distorted picture of what it means to be a Christian. To all who commit their lives into his keeping, Jesus has promised:

~a life that is free from guilt? *True*

~a life that is free from the fear of death? *True*

~a life that can be lived differently with his help? *True*

~a life that is free from sorrow, problems and difficulties? *False*.

Jesus himself was quite blunt about it. 'Here on earth you will have many trials and sorrows,' he said to his disciples, 'but take courage, I have overcome the world.' Being a Christian does not protect anyone from the reality of suffering. We live in a world that is out of harmony with God. Belief is not some kind of spiritual inoculation, which will provide immunity from all that is difficult and painful.

o God cares when we suffer.

In times of crisis it is easy to feel that God is far away and deaf to our cries for help, but this is not so. In the Bible, the prophet Isaiah says: 'In all their distress he too was distressed, and the angel of his presence saved them. In his love and mercy he redeemed them; he lifted them up and carried them.'

This tells me something that I need to hang on to. It assures me that God has not just set the world in motion, seen people mess it up and then left us to get on with it. He is involved. In some way that I cannot fully understand, when I suffer, he, too, suffers. Archbishop William Temple put it like this:

' "There cannot be a God of love," men say, "because if there was, and he looked upon the world, his heart would break."

The church points to the cross and says, "It did break."

"It is God who made the world," men say. "It is he who should bear the load."

The church points to the cross and says, "He did bear it." '

It is supremely in the crucifixion that we see God's identification with human pain; and because of his willingness to suffer there, not just with us but for us and instead of us, we know that his love will not let us down in our darkest hour.

o It is not wrong to grieve.

The prophet Isaiah foretold that the saviour God was going to send would be 'a man of sorrows and acquainted with grief', and Christians see his prophecy fulfilled in Jesus. That does not mean Jesus' life was one long wake – he enjoyed parties and wedding feasts and was criticized for the uninhibited enjoyment of life that he and his disciples displayed. But he also grieved deeply at people's callous and hard-hearted attitudes to one another and at the mess that human rebellion against God had made of the world. He felt human misery so deeply that he worked to the point of exhaustion to heal the sick and reach out to the needy. When his friend Lazarus died, he wept – even though he knew that he was about to cause a sensation by bringing him back to life again. Jesus identified so completely with the despair of the bereaved that he cried with them.

To see someone we love suffering makes us unutterably sad, and God knows that. After all, he gave us our feelings in the first place. But all who come to him need not grieve as 'those who have no hope'. God promises his people comfort and strength right into the valley of the shadow of death, and beyond.

o God is at work in his world.

If God is all-powerful and all-loving, many people ask, why does he allow us to suffer illnesses like cancer? Why does he apparently heal some people – either directly by some miraculous intervention in their lives, or indirectly through medical science (which, after all, he enabled people to discover) – and not others?

This is one of the biggest theological questions of all time, and we will probably never have a completely satisfactory answer in this life. But there are some things we can grasp hold of.

In the beginning of time, the world was perfect and free from any kind of suffering. Human beings spoiled it by choosing to live life their own way rather than God's. Estrangement from God, suffering and death were the inevitable result of this disobedience. God could have abandoned human beings to their fate. Instead he spoke to them constantly, frequently rescued them from the results of their own folly and waywardness, and finally sent his own Son to suffer crucifixion in order to put people right with him. Because of this the power of evil has been broken. God is now at work reconciling men and women to himself, inviting them to join his 'kingdom'. At the moment God's kingdom – his rule in human lives – coexists with the 'kingdom' of this world. While this is so, sin, suffering and death will continue and people can still choose whether to go their own way or God's. Christians believe that one day Christ will return to reign over 'a new heaven and a new earth', where there will be no sin or suffering, no pain or death.

Until this happens, God is at work through people's suffering. Some will be physically healed. Others are given the ability to live with illness and finally to die with trust and hope. Why some are blessed with healing and others entrusted with suffering no one knows. But in either situation, if we will allow him to do so, God will use our suffering for his good purpose. As David Watson said:

'There are seldom good *reasons* for suffering, but there can be good *responses*. I am not suggesting that such good responses are easy. Far from it. For me it has often been an act of the will to listen to worship cassettes, to read the Scriptures, to receive communion, to join in with other Christians, to pray and praise and to meditate on the sufferings of Christ. However, the more I make myself aware of God's love (whether I feel his love or not – usually I don't), the more God can change my negatives into positives. It is a battle, especially at night, but it is certainly important... As we learn to respond positively, however, we shall be able, one way or another, to overcome suffering so that the explanation becomes no longer of major importance. Those who learn that lesson often achieve a remarkable quality of life that may be far in excess of the trouble-free existence of others. It is not what we *do*, but who we *are* that matters most in life; and it is not what we endure but the way we endure it that counts. We can overcome evil with good... For the Christian the future *will* be glorious, and that changes our whole attitude to present suffering. If we think of this world only we have difficulties. But if we see that neither distress nor death can separate us from the love of God, we have a living hope which transcends all the trials of our present existence.'

Those who recognize God's overall control of things in the matter of healing are left with some very practical questions.

o Do we fight the disease or accept it?

Should we encourage the patient to fight or to accept? If it is all in God's hands anyway, does the outcome have anything to do with the way we react?

There are two sides to this particular coin. On the one side is our responsibility to care for our bodies as well as we can. So we can encourage the patient to take the best medical advice that is available, to cooperate with whatever treatment they feel is right, and to help them move towards full health again as positively as we are able.

On the other side is God's ultimate control over life and death – his sovereignty. We acknowledge that the final outcome is in his hands, but that does not mean we cannot pray for healing – either through conventional medicine or by his direct intervention. This prayer may take place privately, between us and God, or publicly, involving others.

Many Christians feel it right to obey the instruction in the New Testament letter of James and, when someone is ill, to 'call the elders of the church to pray... and anoint him with oil in the name of the Lord.' Sometimes this results in actual, provable, physical healing. But even if it does not, the benefits are always felt.

'I was anointed with oil and invited up to the altar rail. Behind me, hands stretched out to rest on my head and touch my back and shoulders and people prayed for me. I don't really remember what they said. I do remember that I prayed a prayer of thanksgiving. I'm told I radiated a light that was overwhelming to people in that sanctuary. They say I was aglow. I know I was aglow with thanksgiving.

'I can't say for sure what happened that day. But I know that

I am alive today, eighteen months later. It is pointless to argue whether the healing I enjoy so far is a result of either medical or spiritual help. I believe it was both. The medical treatments helped my body to fight the cancerous cells. But the laying on of hands – the healing touch – definitely enhanced my emotional needs and nurtured my spiritual self.'

Pat Seed took advantage of the church's sacrament of the Anointing of the Sick when her friend Tony, the then bishop of Lancaster, offered it to her. 'You will either be cured or you will be given the strength to face whatever the future holds for you,' he told her.

'I make no attempt to describe the service. There are some things which are beyond description. It had been truly a sacrament, leaving Geoff and me with greater insight into that familiar phrase, "the peace of God which passes all understanding." The words of the twenty-third psalm took on new meaning, "Though I walk through the valley of the shadow of death I will fear no evil"… suddenly it was all right. The worry was taken away from me and in its place I had peace and a new philosophy. I had been given a job to do. I knew from that moment on that I would be given the strength to do it. What is more, I knew I would not be doing it alone. Cured? I didn't know. It no longer seemed to matter. All that I knew was that I was in God's hands and there was no further need to worry.'

o Whose faith?

In the Gospels, the healing miracles of Jesus are always linked with faith, but it is not always the faith of the person who was ill. There are several instances of friends, employers or parents believing that Jesus could heal and asking him to do so, even if the patient was several miles away. This encourages us to believe that we can pray for another person, whether or not they believe, and God will act – quite often first to awaken in the person concerned a realization of his reality and his love, which is even more important than physical restoration.

And if the patient believes and we do not…? We should not discourage them. After all, if there is 'nothing to it', what harm can be done? And if there is... then maybe it will help us to begin our own pilgrimage of faith.

o What if we pray and nothing happens?

Prayer is never wasted, and something always happens when we pray, although it may not always be exactly what we ask for. We are human and limited in our understanding, and we do not always know how to pray. So the first step before we start praying *for* someone is to ask God what *he* wants to happen in this situation. Sometimes he gives a very clear indication of what he wants to do – through an inner conviction, or a verse from the Bible, or an insight given to another person. When this happens we can pray with confidence, knowing that we are praying 'according to his will'.

At other times we have less certainty and so we can pray only for what seems to us to be the best solution, acknowledging as we do so that God's wisdom is perfect. And we should always pray in cooperation with the patient, for their idea of what should happen and ours may not tally exactly.

'Personally I want people to pray not so much for my healing as for my health. Pray for my holistic health – the "wellness" of my heart, soul, mind and body. Pray also for my acceptance of my condition and that I will have the courage to cope with the consequences of my treatment.'

o What is healing?

There *is* a difference between 'healing' and 'cure'. With only three per cent of medical treatment can a doctor be sure that he can bring about a cure – for the rest, his efforts are directed to helping the body to heal itself.

As we pray and work to help the cancer patient become well again we may reach the point of realizing that healing and cure are not necessarily the same and that a fulfilled life is not always measured in length of years. As Elisabeth Kübler-Ross explains:

'We are not powerless specks of dust, drifting around in the wind, blown by random destiny. We are, each one of us, like beautiful snowflakes that God has created. There are no two snowflakes alike in the whole universe – as there are no two people alike... not even identical twins. Each one of us is born for a specific reason and purpose, and each one of us will die when we have accomplished whatever it was to be accomplished.'

Our view of a completed life is not always the same as God's, and if we do not know how to pray for a cancer patient in terms of a cure, we can pray for healing with confidence. For true healing is not just physical restoration but a completion of God's work in body, mind, emotions and spirit. And that is a prayer that he will surely answer, for he wants each one of us to be whole. And whether the days remaining for us are many or few, he wants us to enjoy rather than endure the time we have left together.

14 A gentle way with cancer

Prince Charles, addressing the British Medical Association on their 150th anniversary, created a considerable stir among the serried ranks of doctors when he suggested that 'the traditional wisdom that sees illness as a disorder of the whole person' was nearer the truth of the matter than a lot of modern medicine would admit. His support of the theory that our health is affected by the way we behave, what we eat and where we live caused ripples of hilarity in some quarters. But more and more people are coming to the point where they can appreciate the wisdom of his remarks, particularly in the case of cancer.

The exact cause of cancer is, of course, still unknown, but there is an increasing body of opinion which agrees with the idea that the development of the tumour is triggered off by damage to the body's defence mechanisms. And this damage can be caused by a number of different factors, not all of them purely physical.

Dr Carl Simonton, Director of the Simonton Cancer Centre in California, says, 'We believe that cancer is often an indication of problems elsewhere in an individual's life – problems aggravated and compounded by a series of stresses 6–18 months prior to the onset of cancer. The cancer patient has typically responded to these problems and stresses with a deep sense of hopelessness... This emotional response, we believe, in turn triggers a set of physiological responses that suppress the body's natural defences and make it susceptible to producing abnormal cells.'

There is no disputing the fact that the physical side of the illness has to be dealt with, and it is usually very well taken care of by the hospital doctors. But cancer is still all too often seen as a purely physical thing by the medical profession, which therefore needs to be dealt with only by conventional medical means. The patients sometimes see things differently.

'My body could not have had better care taken of it at the hospital – I was overwhelmed by their concern for my physical needs. But the worst pain was in my heart and in my mind – and they didn't seem to have any remedies available for that.'

'When I asked the specialist what I could do to prevent a recurrence, he said that there wasn't anything I could do except go home and forget about it until it was time for my next appointment. That was all very well for him – he wasn't sitting at home waiting for the next lump to appear. I felt frustrated and very, very helpless.'

Of course, some patients prefer to be told that they should 'leave themselves in their doctor's hands', and can do so very peacefully and happily. But for many people it is not enough. After all, they reason, if one or more of the physical, mental, emotional and spiritual areas of their lives were involved in their getting cancer in the first place, it makes sense to try and see that, as far as possible, all these areas are now supporting rather than undermining their immune system. They feel that they need all the help they can get as they fight to recover from, or stay clear of, the disease. And this is where the holistic approach comes in.

A sizeable proportion of the population, particularly the medical profession, bristles slightly at the word 'holistic', because it conjures up all sorts of unorthodox (and to their way of thinking 'quack') remedies. This may have been true in the past. It may still be the case with some practitioners in the present – there are charlatans in every branch of medicine. But the word itself is not at all sinister. It is simply taken from the Greek word meaning 'the whole' and implies that the whole person is being taken into account.

Thus, in the holistic view of the disease, cancer is felt to be an illness of the whole system which needs to be tackled on a number of levels. The standard treatment of burning the cancer cells with radiation, poisoning them with chemotherapy or cutting out the definable tumour is seen as probably insufficient on its own to bring about a cure. In addition the body needs to be strengthened by having the right food intake, the mind and emotions need to be freed from anxiety and tensions, and the spirit helped to be at peace with itself, with others and with God, if true health or wholeness is to occur.

So a holistic approach to cancer aims to strengthen:

o the physical – by improving our diet and the level of relaxation and exercise we give our bodies

o the mental, emotional and spiritual – by improving stress control through focusing on greater creativity, positive thinking, meditation and visualization; and by showing people how to be free of guilt, bitterness and other destructive emotions, so that they can experience healing of body and mind.

All these techniques can be seen as complementing, rather than being in any way opposed to, standard medical treatment. Although many doctors would not urge them upon their patients, they would probably not oppose them either, as long as no large outlay of money was involved. The essence of the approach is that it should stimulate self-healing and be totally safe in itself. So, if patients want to experiment with the various techniques, they can do so, knowing that at worst they will do no harm, and at best they may do a great deal of good.

Cancer is a very individual disease and people respond to treatment of all sorts in very different ways. This means that all anyone can do is try to find out what feels right for them, by thinking less in terms of simply curing a disease and more in terms of creating a new and healthier way of living.

Diet
This is the most tangible area to get to grips with, but it is also subject to the most controversy. We have already given some thought to the dietary factors that might be a contributory cause of cancer, but, like everything else in this infuriating disease, a poor diet seems to affect some people adversely and not others. Similarly, some people embark on fruit juice fasts or grape fasts and insist that their cancer has been totally destroyed by such a regime. Others try it and, far from being

made to feel better, are made to feel extremely ill. So is it worth bothering? It would seem that it is, for two reasons.

First, if the patient wants to feel they are doing something positive about their cancer, diet control is relatively easy. It also gives a sense of nourishing and caring for oneself, which is an emotional and psychological benefit.

Second, there is an increasing body of opinion that supports the high fibre, low fat, low salt and sugar way of eating for general good health as well as to give protection against developing a number of diseases. Those who would advocate using diet as a therapy for cancer would suggest a number of variations on this basic theme, or take it several steps further. The general principles seem to be:

o Increase non-animal protein – to the point of adopting a vegetarian diet at least for a few months.

o Eat as much food as possible in its natural state, i.e. not frozen, tinned, preserved or 'interfered with' in any other way.

o Eat as much raw food as possible, concentrating on food which has been organically grown – that is, produced without the use of chemical sprays and fertilizers.

o Use mineral and vitamin supplements where necessary.

The theory behind cutting out meat (and in some cases dairy products as well) is that animals are often fattened by using hormones, and hormones can stimulate the growth of certain cancers. Therefore it is better not to absorb extra hormones into the body via our food. Cutting down on dairy products and red meat will also reduce the saturated fat in our diet, which is held to be a good thing for heart and blood vessels as well as malignant tumours.

The case for 'natural' food is made on the grounds of additives – if some chemicals can be carcinogens, it is not wise to eat food preserved by chemical means when your body's resistance to such things is already at a low ebb. And vitamins are destroyed by cooking, so if you eat more of your food raw, you will increase your vitamin intake without resorting to pills.

All this potential change can seem very threatening and increase tension rather than reduce it, so it is something to be considered carefully and adapted to our own lifestyle. If changes are to be made, they should be introduced gradually (bearing in mind that some people will find it impossible to cope with large quantities of raw fruit and vegetables if they have certain cancers of the digestive tract). It is also very helpful to patients if others in the family will join them in experimenting with this new approach to food – it is much easier to do something different if you are sharing the experience with someone else. And finally we need to remember that the *patient* must want to try this way of strengthening the body's defences, as they must want to sample the other alternative approaches. We cannot force these ideas upon them, however enthusiastic we may feel (nor should we try to deter the patient if we feel less convinced of their potential effectiveness than they do).

Exercise

Some medical practitioners believe that cancer cells do not need oxygen in order to survive, and in fact actually do not like the presence of increased oxygen in the body. If this is so, it would seem that any activity that increases the oxygen intake is a good thing for the patient and a bad thing for the tumour. Other medical experts would dispute this and say that the amounts of oxygen that we can take into the body through normal exercise are not going to make any difference one way or another.

However, whether or not it affects the cancer directly, an increase in aerobic exercise is good for the general health and stamina of patient and relative alike, and if the patient is not well enough to do anything very active to start with, breathing exercises can be a very useful first step. We all know how a few deep breaths can steady the nerves in an anxious situation, and physical activity is a mood lifter as well as an energy booster – unlikely as that may seem when we are tired and depressed. So gentle but increasing activity is something to aim for.

Relaxation

The discovery that you have developed a malignant tumour is quite enough to generate a marked degree of physical and emotional tension. Add to this all the upheaval of treatment, hospital appointments, anxiety about a recurrence of the disease, and all the other worries that are associated with cancer, and it is easy to see why we often feel tense in body and mind. Since stress has been linked with the onset of the disease by many people, both physical and mental relaxation are considered important parts of the 'gentle therapy' for cancer.

Physical relaxation is not the same thing as flopping down in front of the television! Those women and their partners who have attended antenatal classes know that relaxing the muscles throughout the body is a skill that can be learned. But it is a *skill*, and we do not always do it very well the first time we try it. It requires concentrated practice, and it requires time. Both of these can seem very limited when we are struggling to cope with a serious illness. However, it is worth persevering, because not only does relaxation reduce physical stress, it can also be a help in reducing pain – which is why it is used to help a woman in labour.

There are many books and tapes on the market which explain the various relaxation techniques, but, if you want to make a start straight away, you might like to try this simple method.

o Loosen any tight or constricting clothing and find a place where you can remain quiet for about twenty minutes (eventually we aim to be able to relax in the midst of uproar, but you have to make a start somewhere).

o Sit in a chair where you are fully supported with both your feet on the ground, or lie down.

o Focus your concentration on your body and how it is feeling. Start with your feet and consciously relax them, imagining that they are very warm and very heavy. Move on to your lower legs, upper legs and so on through the body, allowing yourself to sink more and more deeply into the chair or bed. Some people find it helpful to tense each part of the body and then relax it, so that they can feel the difference; others do not need to do this.

o Breathe more slowly. Try to feel the air being drawn right down to the bottom of the lungs as you breathe in, and then pushed out in a steady stream as you breathe out. It can be helpful to count as you do this, counting up to four as you breathe in, pausing for a count of two, and then moving on to a count of six as you breathe out, so that the lungs are completely empty. The most important thing is to do it in the way that is comfortable and feels right for you.

And that is a way of gaining physical relaxation. You may not *feel* very relaxed when you try it first, but you can get a good level of relaxation very rapidly if you persevere. What is almost as important, you quickly become aware of the times when you are getting tense, and deal with them straight away.

Stilling the body is one part of relaxation, but it is only partially effective if we have anxious or unhappy thoughts tumbling around in our minds like a hamster on an exercise wheel. We also need to learn how to still the mind, which is usually called 'meditation'.

Meditation
A lot of people dismiss the idea of meditation out of hand, for a variety of reasons. We may feel that:

o it is too difficult

o it is a technique that has sinister implications of brain washing and mind control

o it is not really going to have any bearing on an illness like cancer

o 'I'm not that type.'

While acknowledging that it is not as easy to feel what is happening when we try to still our minds as when we still our bodies, it is possible to measure the effect of mental relaxation and it does have a positively beneficial effect. The big stumbling block to Christians is that many feel that to empty their minds and try to keep them in neutral is to open themselves to the influence of unhelpful spiritual forces, and is not a wise thing to do. I would agree with that, but suggest that the solution is not to avoid the practice, but to focus positively on God.

In the biblical psalms, it repeatedly says:
'I will meditate on your wonders' (Psalm 119:27).
'I meditate on your decrees' (Psalm 119:48).
'We meditate on your unfailing love' (Psalm 48:9).
'I will meditate on all your works... I will remember your miracles

of long ago' (Psalm 77:11, 12).

And the apostle Paul says: 'Fix your thoughts on what is true and good and right. Think about things that are pure and lovely... think about all you can praise God for and be glad about' (Philippians 4:8, Living Bible version).

The mystics of old often used the word 'contemplation' rather than 'meditation', but the basic idea is the same. We need to relax physically first, and then move from the point where our bodies are free from tension and we are breathing gently and quietly, to consciously still the mind. The way in which this is actually achieved varies from person to person. We can learn from others and then experiment until we find something that feels helpful and comfortable to us.

'Just sit down and relax. Slowly and deliberately let all tension flow away and gently seek an awareness of the immediate and personal presence of God... You can relax and let go of everything precisely because God is present. In his presence nothing really matters; all things are in his hands. Tension, anxiety, worry and frustration all melt away before him as snow before the sun... Let your mind, heart and will and feelings become tranquil and serene... "Seek peace and follow after it."'

'When I sit relaxed and breathing quietly I focus on that breathing and picture the atmosphere around me as being full of God's love. As I breathe in, I draw that love into me, and as breathe out I picture all my sadness (or anger, or loneliness) flowing out until it is all replaced by the love (or the peace, or the joy) of God.'

'I kept a tall, fat, red candle and I used to light this. It held no theological significance for me, only a practical one. If my mind was spinning like a top, as it often does, I would watch the flame flicker, listen to the wick splutter and spit, take careful note of the poker-still body and ask God to bring me into that kind of alive stillness.'

'I sometimes think of a verse or phrase from a verse of the Bible, picturing the words in my mind and asking myself what each word or phrase really means to me. Psalm 34:4 is a favourite one.

"I sought the Lord and he answered me; he delivered me from all my fears."

'And I think it through like this:

"I sought" – the personal pronoun – *I* have to look for God for myself, not depend on someone else's experience.

"The Lord" – I'm looking for God, not man-made solutions.

"He answered" – it isn't a fruitless seeking because he answers.

"Me" – it's a personal answer to my personal need.

"He delivered me" – God himself will come to my rescue.

"From all" – he sets me free from *all* – not just some – of the things that trouble me.

"My fears" – I need not be ashamed of my fears – God takes them seriously, but he does not want me to be bound by them.'

'When I lie on the bed, relaxed and warm, I imagine that I am floating in the sea of God's love, held up in it and surrounded by it, rocked gently by the waves. I try to feel the warmth of the sun on my body and imagine that warmth dissolving the cancer cells and pouring in healing.'

All this may sound very strange if you are unfamiliar with the idea of meditation or contemplation, but do not dismiss it out of hand. You do not have to be the 'mystical type' to gain benefit from stilling your mind and opening it to God's presence, and the benefits can be incalculable. The Bible says, 'As a person thinks in his heart, so he is.'

The mind, spirit and body are so closely intertwined that it is just as important to care for the one as it is to look after the other. And, as we quieten our minds, we have a greater ability to get in touch with what is going on under the surface of our lives and to hear God speak to us directly about some of the things which may be acting as a blockage and preventing his healing from working in our experience.

Inner healing
All of us have inner and often deep-seated hurts due to our past experiences. What we may not always consciously realize is that these wounds can leave behind equally deep-seated areas of resentment and bitterness. Until these areas are recalled and specifically dealt with, God's healing process in our lives can be thwarted.

'Kenn explained the importance of thinking of one person at a time, writing down every occasion when I had been hurt by that person. Then I should go through that list... specifically forgiving the individual concerned for each hurt caused, asking God to do the same, praying that God would forgive me for my wrong reactions to those situations, calling on the love of the Spirit to heal those wounds, and finally inviting God to bless the person who hurt me. In this way I could remove any blockages that were still there to God's healing power.'

This forgiveness of others releases us and gives us peace – which is a prime factor in any healing. But there are also times when forgiving others is not enough; we also have to forgive ourselves – and we sometimes find that even harder to do. We give lip service to the fact that God freely forgives all our wrong if we confess it and ask for his forgiveness, but we do not let go of the guilt. We keep it like a stick to beat ourselves with, because unconditional forgiveness seems too much like an easy option. In doing so we devalue what it cost Christ to make that unconditional forgiveness and acceptance possible. Thomas Merton explains it like this:

'We are not permitted to nurse a sense of guilt: we must fully and completely accept and embrace his forgiveness and love. Guilt feelings and inferiority feelings before God are expressions of selfishness, of self-centredness: we give greater importance to our little sinful self than to his immense and never-ending love. We must surrender our guilt and inferiority to him; his goodness is greater than our badness. We must accept his joy in loving and forgiving us. It is a healing grace to surrender our sinfulness to his mercy.'

Put like that, it may sound simple enough. But this kind of soul-searching is often done most effectively with the help of a counsellor who is experienced in the healing of minds and spirits. The church is increasingly aware of the need for this kind of counselling and Christians in many denominations are being trained to help others. If we feel in need of such help, the first person to contact is the minister of the local church. If he is unable to help, or to suggest someone living locally who can do so, there are organizations which offer assistance within a Christian framework.

The forgiveness and healing we have described are not for

Christians only. God's care is for the whole world. Christ died 'for the sins of the world'. Anyone who will may come to him. C.S. Lewis described pain as 'God's megaphone to rouse a deaf world.' And many have indeed sought and found God through pain and suffering.

'Inner healing' or the healing of the mind, emotions and spirit, seems to be the main emphasis in the 'gentle approach' to cancer, but of course we still want to see the physical body restored as well. The Anglican church has a special service of prayer for the sick and, as we have already seen, many people find this very helpful. It may take place through the laying on of hands in the formal setting of a church or as a result of the more informal group of believing friends who simply pray for the person who is ill. Dr Maureen Yates has been helped by both approaches.

'It was Easter 1979 when I first realized that I had developed a lump. I was only thirty-five. Thankfully, I was able to see, quickly, a Christian surgeon in our local hospital. He felt sure that it was only a benign cyst, and arranged to remove it for me two weeks later. After the operation, I was glad that it was he who gently broke the news to me that I had a highly malignant cancer...

'The next day, I read a meditation on Psalm 46 which seemed so appropriate, especially verse 10, which says: "Be still and know that I am God." When I read the comment that "Be still" literally means "Take your hands off. Relax," it seemed an incredible thing for God to be saying to me in that situation, and yet I found myself being able to do just that.

'Emotionally, I was very shaken, and was so glad to be surrounded by my family and friends, some of whom got together to pray specifically for my healing as soon as the seriousness of my illness was realized. Some have been quite certain that God healed me from that moment, despite what was yet to come. Four weeks of radiotherapy treatment were not pleasant, yet despite feelings of nausea and lethargy, there were so many evidences of God's love and care. The shock came towards the end of the treatment, when I discovered that one of my glands was enlarged... Ten days later, at a further small operation, two glands were removed. Both were invaded by cancer. I knew only too well the medical implications for my future, and the outlook certainly looked bleak.

'Just four days after my gland operation, there was a special healing prayer service in my church, and I felt strongly that God wanted me to go forward publicly and ask specifically that Jesus would heal me. Weak in every way, I found it very hard, but I knew that it was a step of obedience. I knew, too, that we were asking for a miracle and nothing less. Afterwards, when asked what I was expecting as a result of that service, I was truthfully able to say that I was expecting God to answer the prayer offered, in faith, by my church, for my complete healing.

'Before commencing a second course of radiotherapy, I was sent away for a week's recuperation. Towards the end of the week, I read Psalm 116:7 in the Living Bible translation: "Now I can relax, for the Lord has done this wonderful miracle for me." It seemed almost too good to be true. At the outset God had told me to relax. Only six days previously I had asked for a miracle. Was this a word from God to me, to believe that he had indeed answered? I looked at the verse in context and found that the whole psalm seemed to describe perfectly my recent experience...

'A year after my first operation, I was dismayed to discover an abnormal patch on my skin. Just to be on the safe side, I went down to the hospital again. I was completely shaken when the radiotherapy consultant told me that he would be very surprised if the skin patch was anything other than a cancer deposit. I could not believe it. Back home, in tears, I felt that God was saying: "Don't let this happy trust in the Lord die away," and "Throw not away your confidence," which to my surprise were both translations of the same scripture verse (Hebrews 10:35). A small group of us prayed, asking God what he was saying to us in this situation. He quite simply reminded us that when God has spoken, that word can never be taken back, but will always be fulfilled...

'Two days later, in a time of worship and prayer with missionary colleagues, God gave me a loving reassurance through impressing these words on the mind of someone I had never met before, saying: "I have made you a promise and I will not fail you. What you have confessed with your mouth and believed in your heart, I will do for you." This was then followed by a worship song, the first verse of which was, "Be still and know that I am God," the second, "I am the Lord that healeth thee," and the third, "In thee, O Lord, do we put our trust." It was yet another instance of the incredible way that everything fitted together, and we knew, as we had already experienced repeatedly, that these were not mere coincidences, but that our God was in control of all things.

'I had to wait a further week for my surgeon to return from holiday, but that quiet peace and confidence which God had given remained with me. The diseased area of skin was removed immediately he returned. Much to the surprise of both consultants there was no evidence of cancer present, and my name was taken off the next day's operating list. God had fulfilled his promise and kept his word.'

One thing which bothers some people is whether we can go on asking for healing if it does not happen straight away. I think that we can if our attitude of heart is right: in other words, if we are simply bringing God our needs, rather than trying to batter him into submission.

Healing is not always instantaneous – even Jesus healed a blind man in two stages on one occasion (the story is recorded in Mark 8:23–25), showing that being freed from illness can be a process as well as one single event. So we can be comfortable about continuing to pray, or asking for prayer more than once. Francis McNutt, who has wide experience of the Christian healing ministry, says:

'One of the great discoveries in my life has been that when a short prayer doesn't seem to help, a "soaking" prayer often brings the healing we are looking for... I have checked the effect of prayer by asking how many were totally healed when we prayed a short prayer and how many were improved. The number of people who experienced some real improvement usually outnumbers those who are totally healed by five to one. This led me to realize that a short prayer usually has some physical effect (and always a spiritual effect) upon a person, but most of us need more time when we pray for the sick.'

Healing, stress control, diet and exercise... here I have tried to give just a bird's eye view of some of the therapies associated with the gentle approach to cancer. Do they matter?

Can they help? Are they effective for the patient alone, or do they have something to offer those of us who are one step removed from the disease itself, but very much involved with our own personal battle to be loving, understanding and supportive? I would say 'yes, they do,' but we must all judge for ourselves.

Cancer is a disease that affects no two people in exactly the same way. It provokes a unique response in each one of us. But, whether we actually have the disease ourselves or are in a supportive role, confronting cancer gives us all an opportunity to discover that there is much more to living than physical health alone. This challenges us to see our needs as a whole, and to work together to meet those needs.

Taking responsibility for your own health and well-being is not an easy option. But for some people it is the best option – the only real way to cope. And, however we choose to handle the crisis that is cancer, we do not have to do it out of our own limited resources.

Penny Brohn, co-founder of the Bristol Cancer Help Centre, put it like this:

'We have to find our own way… The current pattern for dealing with disease is to take it along to an expert and give it to him. Choosing to be responsible for your own illness is not a comfortable position to be in. Less comfortable still is the search to extract meaning from it.

'The search for meaning in suffering is a popular sport amongst religious philosophers and is a bit easier from a library chair than a hospital… but it is a concept worth pursuing. My nervous attempts at this brought me to a place where both the disease and how to cope with it became essentially my problem. I soon discovered that the only person who can carry the weight of this is God… but this has to be Emmanuel – God with us and within us – not a projected fantasy that looks like a cross between Neptune and Tolstoy, glaring balefully down from a cloudy throne. If we are going to know the meaning of "the kingdom of heaven is within you," we must embark on a more intimate relationship with God. Jesus said, "I am the way," and this is the way I have tried to find.'

PART THREE:
The terminal stage

15 The last battle

'There is a time for everything, and a season for every activity under heaven: a time to heal... a time to embrace... a time to be silent and a time to speak... a time to love... a time for peace... a time to weep and a time to laugh... a time to be born and a time to die.'
ECCLESIASTES 3

Cancer is a disease that is often talked about and treated in 'stages'.

The illness can be said to be in its 'initial stage' when the problem is originally diagnosed and treated.

The 'intermediate stage' describes the period covered by remission, which may be partial or complete. During this time the patient is living with the cancer and may remain quite well or may need, and be able to benefit from, intermittent treatment for a period of months or years.

If the disease recurs and then progresses to the point where no further active treatment is available, we speak of the advancing or 'terminal stage'. Death is expected eventually, although again the patient may live for a considerable period of months or even years before this happens.

It is important to understand that a good number of cancer patients have one bout of the disease and eventually die of something completely different. Not everyone will experience the terminal phase of the illness.

As is so often the case with cancer, there is no set pattern. My father probably had his tumour growing for two or three years, but he only *knew* that he had it for twelve weeks – the time that elapsed between his diagnosis and his death. Others have been told that there is no further treatment that would help them and have been in that position for a year, and in some instances considerably longer. So the terminal stage of cancer can last anything from a few days or weeks to a number of years. And if it goes on for a long while, the patient's problems and needs will, initially at least, be much the same as those of anyone who is living with the disease.

Since we have considered those needs in some detail already, we will assume now that the time between the end of active treatment and death is a matter of weeks or months. How can we help the patient (and ourselves) to enjoy, rather than to endure, the life that remains? How can we help them to walk through the valley of the shadow of death with peace and hope?

Practically speaking

A few patients, given the choice, want to return to hospital when their illness progresses, perhaps because they are hanging on to the idea that some miracle cure may yet be discovered. However, most people prefer to be at home and, although those of us who face the prospect of caring for them may doubt our own resources or ability to cope, the basic nursing care is quite simple. There are also professionals at hand to supply what we lack in terms of skill and expert knowledge.

The **local doctor** is usually the first line of support when there is illness in the family, and the terminal stage of cancer is no exception. The patient may have been in hospital for further tests or treatment, or they may have been at home, facing increasing weakness or discomfort, and have been referred back to the cancer specialist briefly for a decision about the future management of the disease. Either way, the specialist will inform the patient's doctor of his findings and make any suggestions about care that he feels are appropriate. If the patient is to be looked after at home, the doctor will then set in motion the wheels of the community care system.

The **district nurse** will renew her contact with the family, and, depending on the family's needs and how far the patient's cancer has advanced, may ask any of the following for help:

o The **health visitor** can offer general support, particularly if the patient is very young or elderly.

o The **physiotherapist** can help in a number of ways to keep the patient mobile, e.g. with walking aids or treatment for swollen limbs or breathing difficulties.

o **Occupational therapists** know where to find gadgets to make life at home easier. They may be able to provide guidance about such things as ramps for a wheelchair or safety devices in the bathroom.

o The **social worker**, often attached to the hospital or local hospice, can give advice on financial problems (and what grants and funds may be available to help cancer patients), home helps, meals on wheels and other voluntary assistance and services. Many are also experienced counsellors who would be glad to listen to any problems that need discussing.

o There are also a number of **specialist nurses** dealing with people suffering from cancer – the Macmillan nurses, the Marie Curie nurses and the hospice continuing care nurses are all experts in the needs of cancer patients, and can be particularly helpful in organizing pain control, making suggestions about diet and being a listening ear for the whole family. The doctor will usually ask them to visit his patient – but if not, we should request him to do so. These nurses work as *advisers*; they do not do 'hands on nursing' – that is the responsibility of the district nurse. There are also **stoma care** and **mastectomy nurses** who can be called in if required, but these will usually have seen the patient in hospital.

If the patient is up and able to get about a little, the need for outside assistance is likely to be less pressing. This situation is the same as nursing anyone who is weak, perhaps in pain and needing a light diet. The four major problem areas tend to be:

o pain

o constipation

o loss of appetite

o sickness and vomiting.

Pain control

Pain *can* be controlled. The most important thing to remember is that the painkillers should be given in sufficiently strong dosages and with enough regularity to keep the patient pain-free at all times. Initially, at least, they are usually given as tablets or in liquid form. If patients are being very sick, the pain relief can be given as suppositories in the rectum (back passage). There are also patches available, rather like those worn by people who want to give up smoking or women on HRT, which release the medication slowly through the skin and are very effective. Less often, people are given a syringe driver which is inserted just under the skin and contains a measured amount of painkiller. This is left in place so that they can press a button and administer a small amount of the drug themselves when the pain is intense.

Apart from specific painkillers, anti-inflammatory drugs can give excellent relief if the patient has secondary cancer in the bones. A course of radiotherapy can also be given for the same reason and is very effective.

It is very difficult for someone who is not feeling pain to evaluate it. It is equally hard for the person suffering from it to describe. Some patients seem to tolerate a great deal without complaint, others appear to have a very low pain threshold. The best rule of thumb is that 'pain is what the patient says it is.' Any pain is important to the person who has it, and should not be taken lightly or ignored. Pain *is* affected by the patient's mood, and someone whose morale is high and whose outlook is positive is likely to be pain-free for longer than the cancer sufferer who is depressed or fearful.

Some carers are anxious about giving too much of a drug in case the patient becomes dependent on it, but there is no need to worry about that in the terminal stage of the illness. As long as we give the prescribed dose and the patient is remaining pain-free and alert, we are doing the right thing. If the pain is returning so quickly that the dosage needs to be increased, or the drugs are causing side effects such as drowsiness, nausea or light-headedness, we should ask the doctor, the district nurse or the specialist cancer care nurse for advice.

Constipation

Painkillers and a low food intake can both provoke constipation. This may seem a very small thing to those who are not suffering from it, but is actually very distressing for the patient. It can in itself also be a cause of pain, so it should not be ignored. The district nurse will suggest a suitable laxative and may also have some helpful ideas about what to eat. Some patients may need to be reassured that a bowel action every day, although desirable, is not essential; two or three times a week is sufficient in this situation. If the problem becomes severe, suppositories and enemas may be given by the nurses.

Loss of appetite

Loss of appetite and subsequent loss of weight is very common with all sorts of cancers and can cause a great deal of anxiety and distress to those of us who are trying to 'build the patient up' and instead see them apparently wasting away before our eyes. The trouble is that a vicious circle can develop, with the patient losing weight, wanting less to eat, losing even more weight, and so on. The principles of care in this area are basically the same as for patients on chemotherapy or radiotherapy.

o Do not press the patient to eat a 'normal' meal – a *little* of whatever they fancy, whenever they feel like eating, will do far more good.

o Small quantities attractively served are more tempting.

o Moist food, possibly liquidized, is easier to swallow.

o Small amounts of alcohol can stimulate the appetite. This is usually all right even if the tablets the patient is taking say 'no alcohol' – as long as they do not drive or use machinery. If unsure, check with the doctor.

o Plenty of plain fluids should be drunk: 8–10 glasses per day if possible.

o Liquids such as soup and ice cream are sometimes more acceptable than solid food and can be enriched with eggs, yoghurt, milk, etc.

o Do not be afraid to discuss any problems with the health care professionals. There are tablets which can be given to improve the appetite and food supplements can also be prescribed.

Nausea and vomiting
If you feel sick you do not want to eat, and if you do eat and are promptly sick the food is not going to do you much good, so this is a problem that needs to be dealt with. The doctor can prescribe anti-sickness drugs which may need to be taken regularly through the day or just half an hour before meals. Other helpful tips worth trying are:

o no fatty or fried foods

o a piece of dry toast or dry cracker biscuit, if eaten immediately after getting up in the morning

o small meals at frequent intervals

o keeping fluid intake and solid intake about an hour apart – do not eat and drink at the same mealtime

o resting immediately before and after eating – but do so sitting up rather than lying flat.

A sore mouth
A dry, sore or infected mouth is another side effect of not eating and drinking properly, and a contributory factor to not wanting to do so. The remedies are the same as for a sore mouth caused by chemotherapy or radiotherapy – very thorough and regular use of the toothbrush, plenty of plain mouth rinses, vaseline for dry lips, plain or flavoured crushed ice to suck, and saliva tablets if the doctor feels they are necessary. If the patient is extremely ill the nurse may use a 'mouth tray' to keep the mouth clean and fresh, but it is much more pleasant if patients can rinse their own mouths for as long as possible. If white patches appear on the tongue, lips and gums, this should be reported to the doctor straightaway as these result from an infection and are very uncomfortable.

Patients should be encouraged to stay up and active for as long as possible, but there will of course come a time when increasing weakness confines them to a chair or their bed for a large part of the time. At this point, unless the bedroom is on the ground floor, the patient and his or her carers will have to decide whether to bring the bed downstairs, so that the patient can still feel part of what is going on in the family, or whether they should be nursed upstairs. There are pros and cons for either situation.

The patient who is nursed downstairs will:

o feel part of the family still

o have more stimulation and interest

o save the carer from running up and downstairs.

But:

o it will be less peaceful and private

o at night the carer will have to sleep downstairs too, possibly in a makeshift bed, or worry that they may not hear and so fail to respond to the patient's call

o there may not be easy access to bathroom and/or toilet.

The patient who is nursed upstairs may:

o feel lonely and isolated.

But:

o will probably have easier access to washing and toilet facilities

o will be able to rest peacefully

o can have a greater degree of privacy when visitors come

o will not be so bothered by food smells if they are feeling sick

o will possibly feel more confident and relaxed at night if the person caring for them is sleeping comfortably nearby.

There is no right or wrong way to handle this. One patient struggled valiantly for weeks to get up and downstairs because, in her culture, to have your bed downstairs was considered to be the beginning of the end (but she did not want to be 'cut off' from her family). The best arrangement to make is the one that feels right to the people most involved – the patient and the person who is caring for them. It is probably wisest for the rest of the family to hold their peace.

Skin care

Once the patient is sitting or lying down for the majority of the time, great care must be taken of the skin – especially that covering bony points such as the heels, elbows, hip bones and the lower back – or pressure sores may develop. The nurse can provide:

o a sorbo rubber ring for the patient to sit on, either in bed or in a chair

o a 'ripple' bed or sheepskin to lie on

o protective padding for heels and elbows

o a bed cradle to keep the weight of the covers off the legs.

All these are aids to prevent pressure, but they are no substitute for helping the patient to change position regularly, and rubbing the pressure points gently with a suitable lotion. (The district nurse will either give you one, or suggest what you should use.) If the skin is dry or itchy, baby lotion is more soothing than talcum powder and does not irritate the lungs. There is a real knack in moving the patient in such a way that it hurts as little as possible, and the district nurse will show you how to do it if asked. Some patients find it helpful and soothing to have their limbs massaged and backs rubbed; others really dislike being touched more than is absolutely necessary. If there are some nursing procedures that the patient really dislikes, it is probably better to leave those, where possible, to the nurses than to create tensions and atmospheres in the family.

As the patient's condition deteriorates the district nurse will visit more and more frequently. She and/or the specialist cancer care nurses will be in daily – if necessary, several times a day – to give injections, blanket baths and other special nursing care. The nurse can arrange for portable toilet necessities such as a commode, bedpan and/or urinal to be provided. If the patient becomes incontinent, she will provide protection for the bed and waterproof padding to keep the patient dry and comfortable. In some areas there is also an emergency laundry service which can help relatives to cope with all the extra washing.

If the urine becomes smelly this should be mentioned, as the patient may have an infection which needs treatment. If the patient develops diarrhoea, this too should be reported to the doctor and, until it is over, fatty and fried foods should be avoided, as should milk products and food with a high roughage content. The patient should not stop taking fluids, however, as severe diarrhoea can lead to dehydration.

The patient as a person
It is easy to be so preoccupied with trying to give the best possible physical care that we lose sight of the person inside the failing body. It is even more important to preserve the dignity of the patient, to help them stay interested in life and contributing to their own care and well-being, than it is to spend hours concocting tempting dishes or ironing sheets.

Time spent reading aloud, listening to the radio or watching television with the patient, doing jigsaw or crossword puzzles, or helping them to carry on with any other sedentary hobby, chatting or simply sitting quietly by the bed is not time wasted but time invested. For enjoying quality of life together involves far more than the most expert or loving physical care.

One day at a time
When we look ahead to weeks, or possibly months, of concentrated nursing we may well feel quite daunted by the prospect and wonder if our resources will last. In our own strength we may well waver, but God has promised that his power is made perfect in our weakness and we can draw on his limitless resources. Jesus summed up an important principle in the Sermon on the Mount when he said to his disciples, 'Don't be anxious about tomorrow. God will take care of your tomorrow too. Live one day at a time.'

When we live like this, we not only refuse to take on tomorrow's worries, we also stop postponing today's small pleasures and savour each day to the full. And since our lives are made up of the sum of our single days, this is the secret of living without regrets or if onlys, whether we are well or ill.

'There are persons who shape their lives by the fear of death, and persons who shape their lives by the joy of life. The former live dying: the latter die living. Whenever I die, I intend to die living...'

No one would pretend, even so, that nursing someone you love through a terminal illness is easy. It is not. However supportive and caring we try to be, there will be times when we get fed up and angry, or feel inadequate and depressed. And when the patient dies we will always be able to look back and find something that we wish we had done differently, something to blame ourselves for. We are human beings, not robots, and human beings do fail. If we demand perfection of ourselves and our relationship with the patient, we shall actually give far less than if we relax and accept that if everyone does the best they can, that is sufficient, and no failure is final – with God.

'God not only forgives our failures; he sees our successes where no one else does, not even we ourselves. Only God can give us credit for angry words we did not speak, temptations we resisted, patience and gentleness little noticed and long forgotten by those around us. Such good deeds are never wasted and not forgotten, because God gives them a measure of eternity.'

Sharing the care

It is also good for both the patient and those caring for him or her to see other people from time to time. We may get over-protective, refusing offers to sit with the patient or take them out for a car ride and feeling that we should be present all the time, but this is a mistake. It is true that some people may overstay their welcome and need to be quietly but firmly removed from the sickroom after a while. It is also true that the patient may not feel able to cope with the over-talkative, or the pessimist, and we may need to stay and help the conversation to remain in the right channels. But this should not stop us from welcoming people who are positive and helpful. We need to use such times to give ourselves a much-needed break from the constant care.

In every nursing situation there are one or two people who bear the major responsibility for the patient's care, and others who help when they can. Tensions can arise within a family when those who are in the reserves try to interfere with the pattern that the first team has established.

Stephen's father lived in the same area as his son. When his cancer became very advanced, Stephen's sister put pressure on her father to leave his flat and move in with her brother. She herself lived 100 miles away and worked full-time, which Heather, Stephen's wife, did not. But Heather found it hard to cope with her three young children and a very sick father-in-law. She found it even harder to endure her sister-in-law's fortnightly visits. Jean stayed in her father's flat, but expected to eat all her meals at her brother's home and, instead of helping with her father's care and allowing Heather and Stephen a little free time, constantly criticized the way in which he was being nursed.

This situation was eventually resolved when the doctor told Jean very firmly that he was admitting the patient to the local hospice to establish better pain control and to give the family a rest. He also suggested that she should address any further comments or complaints to him.

The principle to be observed in this situation is that the reserves should support and encourage. If they have any queries or comments about the treatment, the nursing care, or the course that the patient's illness is taking, they should go directly to the medical care team rather than undermining the confidence of the rest of the family.

16 Together through the valley

Dying can be seen not merely as the end of life but as a very special phase of personal growth and development. However, almost everyone would hear the words, 'I'm afraid there is no more treatment that will help,' with an initial sense of foreboding, if not with downright panic. We may come to accept the inevitability of death, but we are hardly likely to relish the prospect in the foreseeable future, however firmly we may believe that death is not the end. David Watson, strong man of faith though he was, was no exception.

'My immediate reaction was to think that I had roughly 365 days more, so the next day it was only 364, then 363. This proved to be both depressing and crippling in its negative effect. I had always imagined that for those under sentence of death the worst experience was probably not the sentence itself but the agonizing period of waiting. Every morning you wake up with the same nightmare that does not fade with the day, since it is reality. Every night the same dreams haunt you. Imagination loves to feed on fear and the result can be almost paralyzing...

'The worst times for me were at two or three o'clock in the morning. I had preached all over the world with ringing conviction. I had told countless thousands of people that I was not afraid of death since through Christ I had already received God's gift of eternal life. For years I had not doubted these truths at all. But now the most fundamental questions were nagging away... If I was soon on my way to heaven, how real was heaven? Was it anything more than a beautiful idea? What honestly would happen when I died? Did God himself really exist after all? How could I be sure? Indeed how could

I be certain of anything apart from cancer and death? Never before had my faith been so ferociously attacked.'

David was one of those cancer sufferers whose disease had spread too far for active treatment before he even suspected that he had it. So he and his family had to cope with all the emotional trauma of coming to terms with the diagnosis *and* accepting that his life might shortly be coming to an end, at one and the same time.

Other people may have worked their way through the stages of grief after the diagnosis and consider that they have accepted the fact of having cancer. They then feel shocked and disappointed because the denial, anger, depression or bargaining all flood back again, and have to be faced once more, when death comes closer. There is no set order or pattern in which this occurs – it is rather like the tide coming in and depositing its flotsam and jetsam on the beach. One morning, as we walk along the tide line, we may find seaweed and driftwood; on another occasion we may discover bits of rope, oil or empty tins and bottles; and after the next tide all may be swept away again and the sand left clear and unspoiled.

This would seem to be true of the emotions that patient and family alike may experience during the terminal stage of cancer. One day anger or bitterness may come flooding in, but on the next tide hope and acceptance may sweep them away. It helps to understand this, because we may not all work through the identical stage of grief at the same time. The tide may be washing acceptance over the patient's 'beach' and swirling depression onto mine. Some people seem to react in the opposite way from one another, whereas others are much more influenced by the emotional current surrounding them and get swept along together. Neither response is better or worse than the other – we just need to recognize what is happening and bring all our resources of patience and understanding to bear on the situation.

'I thought that I had beaten cancer in my mind and my emotions, if not in my body. But when the doctor said that he could do no more, the struggle started all over again.'

Apart from the feelings associated (and sometimes intertwined) with grief, the cancer patient has other emotional pitfalls which they may stumble into.

Guilt

Taking responsibility for your own illness and working hard to maintain a positive outlook are very good attitudes, but if the cancer recurs in spite of their best efforts some patients feel very guilty. They may blame themselves for not trying hard enough or not following a particular course of treatment with sufficient care. If they have had prayer for healing, they may worry that they did not have 'enough faith' or that there is some unrecognized and unconfessed wrongdoing in their lives which has prevented God's healing power from working.

Most people recognize that their illness does put a great deal of stress and strain on the people caring for them, and may feel guilty about that, and some even feel guilty because they imagine that they have let their family down by not recovering.

This guilt is often not dealt with, because it is not expressed – at least not in so many words. So the first team supporters need to be sensitive to this particular area of suffering and assure the patient that it is not their fault if the disease returns and they need extra care. To look after one another is the privilege and prerogative of loving, but we often find this hard to put into words. We may imagine that our actions speak loudly enough, but in fact words *are* needed and can bring a great deal of comforting reassurance. And where there is guilt and remorse over past misdeeds or broken relationships, 'sorry' also needs to be said and received with openness and love.

One of the great cornerstones of the Christian faith is that all the wrong we have ever done can be forgiven *and* forgotten if we are willing to bring it to God. But we sometimes find it difficult to admit a need, or to help someone close to us to understand that. This is where an outsider can be of great help. Some ministers offer the opportunity for formal confession within the framework of the church; others would be glad to listen and offer comfort and assurance in a more informal setting. Unfinished business of this kind can be a great source of pressure to the seriously ill patient, and has a considerable potential for causing unnecessary grief and regret to those who survive him, so it is important to get it dealt with in whatever way is appropriate to our situation.

It is never too late to find peace with God, or to make peace with those we have wronged.

Loneliness

There is an awful finality about being told that nothing further can be done to treat your disease, and patients often feel abandoned by their doctor at this point. The doctor (for reasons already discussed) may increase this sense of isolation by withdrawing slightly and appearing to lose interest in someone whom he or she cannot hope to see return to health again. Friends too may feel uncomfortable and uncertain how to handle the situation, and so avoid contact. Loneliness can be intense.

'I began to wonder whether my wife was secretly longing to be free of me too, and felt a bit like Jesus when he said to the disciples, "Will you also go away?" The trouble was that I could not ask the question, because I felt that to do so was to put her in the position of *having* to say no. It was a tremendous relief – like a light being switched on in the darkness – when she said one day, "We'll see this through together, no matter what happens." '

Fear

Death is the one certainty in life which everyone shares, and yet we all tend to ignore it for as long as we can. But, in the famous words of Samuel Johnson, 'When a man knows that he is to be hanged in a fortnight, it concentrates his mind wonderfully.' And when we are faced with a shortage of future, we become aware of questions which can no longer be shelved or ignored.

Even the most steadfast believers are likely to re-evaluate the foundations of their faith at such a time. Some prefer to do it quietly; others need to debate and discuss with someone who will not be shocked by this apparent wavering.

Many have never really crystallized what they do believe. Although they might be embarrassed to admit a need for inner certainty, they may be thankful for an opportunity to talk things through. (For helpful books in this area see the book list on page 186.) For research has shown that it is those who have their beliefs sorted out who are able to face the future without fear – whether they believe that death is the end, or that it is the beginning of something more wonderful than we can ever imagine. The waverers in the middle have a rather tougher time.

Although many people say that they do not fear death itself, the process of dying is another matter. The word cancer is closely linked with pain in many people's minds, and one of the greatest fears that patients have is of a lingering and extremely painful death. Fortunately, in these days of ever increasing understanding about pain control, at least half of the patients who have advancing cancer have no significant pain at all, and for those who do, very effective relief is available. Reassurance on this front can and should be given by the doctor, the district nurse, or the specialist cancer care nurses who are becoming more commonly available to enable the patient to be cared for comfortably at home.

For those of us who are doing the caring, it is helpful to know that pain is often linked to emotional distress. This is not a reason to tell the patient that their pain is 'all in the mind', but an encouragement to give them the support that they need, so that this distress factor can be alleviated. For those who doubt their ability to cope with watching those they love suffer, it is also cheering to note that pain, even very severe pain, is rarely remembered by the patient once it is over.

'I cannot recall the pain. I can remember having the experience of intense pain, but not the pain itself. I thank God I can't; otherwise life would be unbearable. I can recall it now only as an abstract concept.'

One other area of fear that both the patient and relatives may share is how those left behind will cope with the future. It is difficult to speak about these things openly, but a great relief to both sides when it is done. If the carers want, the doctor, district nurse, minister or a more distant relative or close friend can introduce the subject of a will, financial arrangements for the future, or perhaps whether it is wise to spend money on the house. In this way they can act as a catalyst. These are some of the things that need to be discussed:

o The will. If the patient dies without making one, it makes life unnecessarily complicated for the surviving relatives.

o Guardians or trustees for any dependent children.

o Financial provision – insurance, pensions, etc.

o Whether the patient has any particular wishes about the funeral; whether they want to be buried or cremated, or even to donate their body or organs to medical research.

Some patients have very definite ideas about what form they want their funeral service to take, and go as far as working out their own order of service with their choice of hymns and readings. This can be hard to talk about at the time. But it is immeasurably comforting afterwards to know that everything has been done as the patient wanted. However, we should not try to force such participation, unless the patient really wants it.

Helplessness

If a medical expert says he can do no more for you, there is a considerable temptation to think that you can do no more for yourself either, and this can lead to a feeling of utter helplessness. However, this need not be the case, as many cancer sufferers have proved when they have turned to alternative forms of medicine at this very point in their lives. In addition to doing what suits them in those 'gentle' ways that we have already considered, patients should be encouraged to set their own goals and to discover for themselves what they can and cannot cope with, rather than being dictated to by anxious relatives.

In 1983 an American group who aimed to help the Christians in poorer countries to preach and teach their fellow countrymen about their faith received a request from a Filipino evangelist for 100,000 New Testaments. He assured them that he intended to distribute these within the next six months. This seemed to be a very large undertaking and the Americans, anxious to ensure proper use of the supplies, delayed sending the books until they had made a few enquiries.

They elicited the fact that the man had distributed 100,000 Testaments in the previous six months, even though he had no means of transport other than a backpack with which to carry them. Whilst they still debated whether they should fulfil his request for further supplies, a friend of the evangelist wrote and pointed out that two months had been wasted and the matter was *urgent*.

'Why is the need so pressing?' they asked. The reply came by return: 'The evangelist is eighty-one years old and has terminal cancer. He has been given six months to live.'

Obviously he was an exceptional man, with an unusually high degree of motivation. But, although few people in his position would set themselves such an ambitious goal, many have made up their minds that they will *live*, not just exist, until they die, and have done so with considerable success. As Sandra Grantstrom, an American nurse, once wrote: 'A reason must be found for living with the limitations of the illness or the patient will not. In this quest, all human beings must have something to believe in, something to hope for and someone to love and to return their love.'

Another antidote to the paralysis of helplessness is to encourage the patient to make their own decisions for as long as they are able to do so. This means that *they* decide (if there is an option) whether they wish to be nursed at home, in hospital or in a hospice. Of course, there will be times when there is no choice, because there is no one to care for the patient at home, or their condition necessitates the facilities of a hospital or hospice. But we should make sure that the options are discussed and not jump to conclusions too quickly.

Tony's mother lived alone and at a distance from him and, when her cancer became advanced, Tony insisted that she came and lived with him – out of the kindest of motives. The elderly lady moved reluctantly and was utterly miserable away from her friends and familiar surroundings. Eventually she returned home to be cared for by the district nurse and the local Macmillan cancer care nurses who visited her daily, and even more frequently as her illness progressed. She managed to stay at home until ten days before she died. At that point she was admitted to the local hospice. It may seem a very lonely course of action to have pursued, but it was what *she* wanted and she was happy and peaceful to the end.

This right to decision-making should also be extended to the situation where treatment is achieving very little and the patient wants to stop having it. This happens most commonly with chemotherapy, but it can also occur when radiotherapy or further surgery may prolong life a little, but offer the patient a very poor quality of life in return for the extra time. The patient often feels obliged to keep on with the treatment for the sake of the family, and the family hesitates to encourage them to stop because it may hasten the end of their life.

'My mother was having chemotherapy for one week out of every four, so that the tumour on her jaw did not grow any larger. The problem was that she felt really ill for perhaps two out of the three non-treatment weeks – her life was really miserable, and there was no hope of a cure. She had said in a "down" moment that she did not want any more treatment, but I knew that she would not say so to the doctor, so I went along with her for her next appointment and asked some questions that brought the whole thing out into the open. The doctor suggested that she should have a three-month break and then reconsider.

'When the three months were up we went back to the hospital again and my mother asked what would happen if she did not have any further treatment. The doctor simply said, "The tumour will grow," and left us for ten minutes or so (in the hospital corridor) to make our decision. I told her that whatever she decided, I would support her in that decision, and that she did not have to struggle on with the chemotherapy for my sake. Once she had reassured herself that I would still visit her as often as before if she was not having the treatment, she relaxed visibly and told the doctor her decision quite calmly. I sometimes wonder if I did the right thing, but I know that she enjoyed the last six months of her life far more than the previous eighteen, and that is the most important thing.'

These, then, are some of the fears that patients and their families face. Each situation varies and the thing that is immensely important to one person may not raise a ripple of disquiet for another. All we can do, in trying to help, is to attempt to identify the particular stress that is bothering the patient *at that moment*, and then try to respond to the emotions and needs expressed. This may mean offering practical help, or emotional or spiritual support. The important thing is that we do not try to impose our expectations of how patients should react, but endeavour to meet them where they really are, rather than where we think they should be.

Letting go
There is a very fine line between encouraging the patient to fight the disease and allowing them to let go of their hold on life.

Joe was content to 'go right through the valley', as he put it, but he felt as if his wife Edith was holding back.

'She keeps reminding me of all that we planned to do when we retired,' he said wistfully, 'but I know and she knows that those plans were shelved a while ago. She wants me to fight... but I've no more fight left in me... and yet I can't let her down!'

It is hard to admit that your life is drawing to a close, and some people never do, but most patients gradually withdraw from life, want to see fewer people and slowly lose interest in the wider world. This is not 'giving up', but part of the natural process. We can help or hinder the peacefulness of this stage by our attitude.

Edith finally acknowledged to Joe that her future would be faced without him, and together they dealt with the unfinished business of where she would live, how she would manage financially and what part of their former plans she would be able to carry out alone. When they had done this, they were both able to see Joe's life as completed, and he died peacefully two or three weeks later, knowing that he had done all that he could to care for his wife's needs.

If we decide to nurse the patient at home right through to the end of their life, it is usually possible to do so. But in some cases it is necessary for the patient to be admitted to hospital for some specialist nursing care, or to spend time in a hospice for pain control, or simply to give the family a rest. If this happens, we should not blame ourselves or feel that we have failed.

'I couldn't possibly allow my husband to be taken to a hospice – he would think that I had deserted him.'

'Won't a hospice be a very dreary place to end her days? It must be very gloomy... so full of dying people.'

If we have never been to a hospice it is easy to share the feelings expressed by those two anxious relatives, but their fears have no foundation in fact. Hospices usually have a very happy, peaceful and loving atmosphere, and are not at all gloomy or depressing. Although they specialize in the care of the terminally ill, many patients go there for short periods and come home again, and by no means all the people there are at death's door. Added to this, the staff are trained in the care of cancer patients. They are experts in pain control and in the needs of those whose lives are ending – and of their families.

The whole philosophy of hospices is very positive – to support and encourage those who are terminally ill, and to enable them to face death when it comes with courage, dignity and hope. And, although the reality of the patient's situation is not brushed aside, the emphasis is on *living* – living with the minimum of pain and discomfort – making every day that remains the very best it can be, within the limits of the individual's physical condition. So visitors are encouraged; children and even family pets are usually welcomed, and most patients are kept active and cheerful.

Some hospices have teams of nurses who visit patients in their homes and give support and advice where it is needed. So it is not an admission of defeat to call on the resources of our local hospice. If we have never had any contact previously, it can be a good idea to telephone and ask to pay the hospice a visit, long before there may be any need for us to avail ourselves of the help that is offered. Before a patient can actually be admitted to the hospice, the doctor has to complete a referral form. But most continuing care centres, as they are sometimes called, welcome a direct enquiry from the family. They provide a great deal of support for families too, both during the patient's illness and after his or her death.

Death and dying

Few people these days have ever come into direct contact with death – it is a process which, like birth, more often occurs within the clinical confines of the hospital. So it is natural for us to be uneasy at the prospect of our loved one dying at home, even though we may really want them to be where they are happiest and feel most at peace. Most of the fear is fear of the unknown, however, and so we should not hesitate to ask the doctor or district nurse anything that we want to know about the final stages of the illness.

One of the major things that we may feel concerned about is how we will know when death is near. We may wish to alert other members of the family, or to ensure that the husband or wife, or other chief carer, is not left to care for the patient alone at this time. Unfortunately, it is not possible to give exact guidelines, because once again people vary as much in the way they die as the way they live with cancer. But there are some things we can be sure about:

o Death rarely happens suddenly when patients are suffering from cancer – we will usually have some warning that their condition is deteriorating because they will sleep more, and often drift from sleep into unconsciousness, from which they cannot be roused. The pattern of breathing also changes, and may become noisy, which is distressing to hear, but is simply caused by moisture in the chest.

o By the time the patient is as ill as this, we will be receiving daily or even more frequent visits from the district nurse, and she will be able to confirm our fears, or reassure us that death is not yet imminent.

o Although the patient may not be able to say anything and appears to be unconscious, the sense of hearing is the last sense to be lost. So they can still appreciate and be comforted by words – expressions of our love, favourite Bible readings or prayers, or well-loved music.

o People dying from cancer are most unlikely to writhe in agony or show any other untoward signs of distress, as some relatives fear. For the vast majority of people it is a gentle process – they fall ever more deeply asleep and eventually simply stop breathing.

Practicalities

The first thing we need to grasp is that a dead body is nothing to be afraid of. It is simply the empty and now unneeded shell of the person we have loved – rather like the shrivelled chrysalis from which a beautiful butterfly has emerged. When the heart stops beating and the breathing stops, the body becomes very pale and gradually colder.

It is not necessary to do anything to the body at this time, and no one will think any less of those who do not wish to do so. However, many people who have been closely involved in the patient's care feel comfortable about straightening the body, removing all except one pillow, closing the eyes if that is needed and supporting the jaw with a pillow or book. Any heating in the room can be turned off. In these days there is rarely anyone in the community who is the official 'layer out', and in fact the process is much simpler than it used to be. If we wish to do so it is quite in order to wash the person's face and hands and put clean night clothes on them, but that is entirely up to us. The undertaker will care for this side of things if we do not feel able to do so.

The doctor is the first person to be informed, and the body cannot be removed from the house until he has certified that death has taken place. Even if the patient dies during the night, the doctor will usually come straight away, and then it is up to us whether or not we wish the undertaker to remove the body immediately or to wait until the morning, or later in the day. Many people would not wish to wait, but others prefer to allow the rest of the family to arrive and say their goodbyes in private. Especially if there are children closely involved who wish to see the body, it is often easier for them to accept the reality of death, without fear, if they see their parent or grandparent lying peacefully in their own bed, rather than in the more unnatural setting of the funeral home.

Those of us who are part of a local church will have our own minister to whom to turn at this time. He will come and offer comfort, care and help with all the arrangements that have to be made for the funeral. The funeral director will also make a return visit to the family, probably within twenty-four hours of the death taking place, so that the practical details of the burial or cremation can be worked out. If the family have no firm ties with a place of worship, he will also be able to make suggestions about the form of the funeral service and liaise with the cemetery chapel and the minister who is on duty there, if this is what the relatives wish to happen.

The funeral

Many of us dread the prospect of the funeral and almost wish that it need not take place, but it is actually a very important stage in the process of grieving, and helps us to come to terms with what has happened. It is a public declaration of what has taken place, encourages us to 'let go' of the person who has died and enables us to thank God for them. It is also a time when we can gather a great deal of strength and comfort from the love and support of our wider family, close friends and the community in which we live.

'I did not want a miserable funeral. I wanted a triumphant thanksgiving for Don's life – his courage, his care for others and his indomitable spirit. I suppose I also felt I had to put a brave face on if I believed (as I did... and still do) that, far from being dead, he was triumphantly and vigorously alive in another dimension. So when I burst into tears at the graveside I felt as if I was letting God down.'

Ann expressed the very mixed emotions that Christians feel when faced with death. Yes, we do believe that death is not the end, and that what lies beyond this life is far better than anything that we have enjoyed thus far. But we are still experiencing loss on a massive scale when we are parted so completely from someone we love, and tears are not a sign of weakness or lack of faith. If Jesus wept when he knew that Lazarus' resurrection was only moments away, we can certainly do so too.

Even those who believe in life after death still grieve – for themselves if not for the one who has died – because there are no short cuts through mourning, and any death, whether sudden or long expected, is shocking and devastating in its finality. But in all the sadness – although others may appear to forget and pick up the threads of their lives once more, and we may feel out of step with an uncaring world – we will find that we can depend utterly on God's total understanding, unfailing comfort and limitless love. And eventually the darkness *will* give way to the dawn. We *will* come to terms with the questions, the pain and the loss, and with a new understanding and absolute assurance we shall be able to say, 'I know that nothing is mightier than God – not the severest hardship, nor the deepest distress. His power to help is always greater.'

Afterword

'Let there be new beginnings.'

When my father slipped quietly out of this life into life eternal, his encounter with cancer had ended and mine had just begun. While I grieved and struggled to make sense of it all, I talked to many people who have also come face to face with cancer. Their experiences, their questions, their confusion, their certainties and their courage have been woven together to form the basis of this book. To all of them I have put the question, 'What have you learned ... what difference has this confrontation with cancer made to your life?' Some of their answers you have already read.

I thought after my father's illness that I had got a handle on it all, until three and a half years ago, when I had to face the fact that the dark shadow of cancer had been cast across our family once more. Then I realized that I had to work my way through to peace and acceptance all over again. My husband is well at present, but we have to accept that he is living with the disease and we do not know what the future may hold. We haven't found that easy. But we can both say with confidence that facing the reality of death has given us a whole new perspective on our life together. We have proved that although the path through the valley of the shadow is dark and difficult, although grief and fear may tear at our hearts and doubt may threaten to send us headlong, God always goes before, to prepare the next step. Not only that, he also comes behind to gather us up and carry us when we have felt too weary to face another step. And as he lifts us up, he also collects our sadness and our mistakes, the opportunities taken and missed, our achievements and our failures, so that none of them is wasted and all can be used for our good, because God is in the business of new beginnings. And what he has done for us, he is ready and willing to do for everyone who turns to him in their need.

Now that I have struggled back to the place where this certainty is once again a tried and tested rock beneath my feet, I can step out with renewed confidence and a wider perspective on life and death. If life is such a fragile and fleeting gift, I want, more than ever, to experience it fully before I die. I want to live trustingly, so that I will have no fear of the present or the future. I want to live lovingly with others, so that when I reach the end of my journey there are no regrets or if onlys. I want to live so that every day has quality, no matter what quantity of time is allotted to me or to those whom I love. I want to live wisely, so that I can know what is truly worth the investment of my time. And most of all I want to serve the purpose of God in my generation. This realization is the treasure that coming face to face with cancer has unearthed for me – and yes, it is worth the price.

Book list

Personal experience

Penny Brohn, *Gentle Giants*, Century Hutchinson
Fiona Castle and Jan Greenough, *No Flowers… Just Lots of Joy*, Kingsway Communications
Rachel Clyne, *Coping with Cancer*, Harper Collins
Brenda Courtie, *A Year on the Sofa*, obtainable from the author at The Baptist Manse, Stoke St Gregory, Taunton TA3 6JG; £6.00 including postage and packing
David Watson, *Fear No Evil*, Hodder and Stoughton

Personality and stress

Carl and Stephanie Simonton, *Getting Well Again*, Bantam Books

Meditation

Joyce Huggett, *Listening to God*, Hodder and Stoughton

The modern hospice movement

Shirley Du Boulay: *Cicely Saunders*, Hodder and Stoughton

Emotional issues

Elisabeth Kübler-Ross, *To Live Until We Say Goodbye*, Prentice Hall
Elisabeth Kübler-Ross and David Kessler, *Life Lessons: Two experts on death and dying teach us about life itself*, Simon and Schuster

Specific cancers

Tom Smith, *Coping Successfully with Prostate Cancer*, Sheldon Press
Jonathan Waxman, *The Prostate Cancer Book*, Vermilion
Roger S. Kirby, *The Prostate: Small gland, big problem*, The Prostate Research Campaign

Other resources

Eleanor Meade with Rosemary Conley, *Facing Breast Cancer: Questions about breast cancer and post-operative exercises*, Compassion Productions Ltd; tel. 01303 210250

Fight Back and Get Fit, an information and exercise video featuring Rosemary Conley and Eleanor Meade for pre- and post-operative breast cancer patients, obtainable from Christian bookshops or direct from Compassion Productions, PO Box 430, Folkestone, Kent CT20 2GP; www.compassion.co.uk; e-mail: mail@compassion.co.uk

Eleanor Meade's story of her experience of breast cancer is also obtainable on CD. Entitled *What If*, it is free to any woman who has breast cancer. Also available from Compassion Productions.

Useful addresses

There is a huge amount of information about cancer on the internet. Some of it is reliable, some of it is not. Always check with your doctor before implementing any advice given.

General cancer information

www.iconmag.co.uk

www.cancerlinks.org, a website designed to make searching the internet easier

Cancer Research UK provides a free information service called CancerHelp UK on all aspects of cancer for patients and their families. Cancer Information Nurses are available on freephone 0800 226237. More information can be found at www.cancerresearchuk.org and www.cancerhelp.org.uk.

CancerBACUP, 3 Bath Place, Rivington Street, London EC2A 3JR. A team of experienced cancer nurses will deal with written and telephone queries on all aspects of cancer care; tel. 0808 800 1234; www.cancerbacup.org.uk. They publish a number of useful booklets.

Macmillan Cancer Relief; tel. 0808 808 2020; www.macmillan.org.uk

Marie Curie Cancer Care, 89 Albert Embankment, London SE1 7TP; tel. 020 7599 7777; www.mariecurie.org.uk

St Christopher's Hospice, Lawrie Park Road, Sydenham, London SE26 6DZ; tel. 020 8768 4500; www.stchristophers.org.uk

The Leukaemia Care Society, 2 Shrubbery Avenue, Worcester WR1 1QH; tel. 01905 330003 or 0845 767 3203; www.leukaemiacare.org

The British Colostomy Association, 15 Station Road, Reading, Berkshire RG1 1LG; tel. 0118 939 1537; www.bcass.org.uk

Breast cancer

Breast Cancer Campaign, Clifton Centre, 110 Clifton Street, London EC2A 4HT; 020 7749 3700; www.bcc-uk.org

Breast Cancer Care, Kiln House, 210 New Kings Road, London SW6 4NZ; tel. 020 7384 2984; www.breastcancercare.org.uk

UK Breast Cancer Coalition, c/o Breakthrough Breast Cancer, 3rd Floor, Kings Way House, 103 Kingsway, London WC2B 6QX; tel. 020 7405 5111; www.ukbcc.org.uk

Lung cancer

The British Lung Foundation, 73–75 Goswell Road, London EC1V 7ER; tel. 0207 688 5555; www.britishlungfoundation.com

Prostate cancer

The Prostate Cancer Charity offers telephone advice from trained nurses 10.00–4.00 Monday–Friday; tel. 0845 300 8383; www.prostate-cancer.org.uk.

Complementary services

The Haven Trust; tel. 0207 384 0000; www.thehaventrust.org.uk

Index